Negotiating nursing

MANCHESTER
1824

Manchester University Press

Nursing History and Humanities

Series editors: Christine E. Hallett and Jane E. Schultz

This series provides an outlet for the publication of rigorous academic texts in the two closely related disciplines of Nursing History and Nursing Humanities, drawing upon both the intellectual rigour of the humanities and the practice-based, real-world emphasis of clinical and professional nursing.

At the intersection of Medical History, Women's History and Social History, Nursing History remains a thriving and dynamic area of study with its own claims to disciplinary distinction. The broader discipline of Medical Humanities is of rapidly growing significance within academia globally, and this series aims to encourage strong scholarship in the burgeoning area of Nursing Humanities more generally.

Such developments are timely, as the nursing profession expands and generates a stronger disciplinary axis. The MUP Nursing History and Humanities series provides a forum within which practitioners and humanists may offer new findings and insights. The international scope of the series is broad. It embraces all historical periods and includes both detailed empirical studies and wider perspectives on the cultures of nursing.

Previous titles in this series:

Mental health nursing: The working lives of paid carers in the nineteenth and twentieth centuries
Edited by Anne Borsay and Pamela Dale

One hundred years of wartime nursing practices, 1854–1953
Edited by Jane Brooks and Christine E. Hallett

'Curing queers': Mental nurses and their patients, 1935–74
Tommy Dickinson

Histories of nursing practice
Edited by Gerard M. Fealy, Christine E. Hallett and Susanne Malchau Dietz

Nurse Writers of the Great War
Christine Hallett

Who cared for the carers? A history of the occupational health of nurses, 1880–1948
Debbie Palmer

Colonial caring: A history of colonial and post-colonial nursing
Edited by Helen Sweet and Sue Hawkins

NEGOTIATING NURSING

BRITISH ARMY SISTERS AND SOLDIERS IN THE SECOND WORLD WAR

JANE BROOKS

Manchester University Press

Published by Manchester University Press
Altrincham Street, Manchester M1 7JA
www.manchesteruniversitypress.co.uk

British Library Cataloguing-in-Publication Data
A catalogue record for this book is available from the British Library

ISBN 978 1 5261 1906 3 hardback

First published 2018

Typeset by Servis Filmsetting Ltd, Stockport, Cheshire
Printed by Lightning Source

This book is dedicated to my mother, Margaret Brooks,
and in memory of my aunt, Pam Brooks.

Contents

Figures

Acknowledgements

I should like to thank the Queen Alexandra's Royal Army Nursing Corps and their Heritage Association for supporting this project. My thanks also goes to the History of Nursing Society of the Royal College of Nursing Foundation, for their support through the Monica Baly Bursary and to the Wellcome Trust whose early support for *One Hundred Years of Wartime Nursing Practices* (Manchester University Press, 2015), acted as a valuable precursor to the work for this book. I am also very grateful to the following archives, libraries, museums and their staff for preserving the documents and oral histories used in this monograph and for making them available: the Museum of Military Medicine, the Imperial War Museum, the Wellcome Trust Library and Archives, the Royal College of Nursing Archives, the British Library, the National Archives and the archives of the Princess Mary's Royal Air Force Nursing Service. I have used extensive quotations from several of these archives and these and other personal testimonies have formed the backbone to my research. My thanks and appreciation for all that you have done to make this book possible. I should also like to thank the Museum of Military Medicine for permission to use all the images used in the book and on the front cover. This was a most generous gift and I am truly grateful.

I should like to offer my profound thanks to all the retired nurses who gave their time to support this project. Their contributions have been critical to the ideas in *Negotiating nursing*, whether or not I was ultimately able to use their testimonies. I am also indebted to those who supported these women to be able to provide their memories. Families and friends of nursing sisters have generously provided diaries, memoirs and recollections. Many of these have not been published before and have therefore enabled this book to include highly original primary source material. My great thanks go to the following: Rowena Quantrill, Barbara Collins' daughter for providing me with access to her mother's letters home; Nell Jarrett's nephew and niece, Phillip John and his sister Chris, and Phillip's wife, Anna John, for providing me with full access and permission to use Sister Jarrett's diary, press cuttings and photographs; Liz Williams for the reminiscences of her mother, Winifred Mountford (Monty), who served with the QAs in the UK, northern France and Egypt during the Second World War; Penny Salter's friends for providing me with full access to her diary and the various press reports of her wartime nursing experiences; and Jessie Wilson's family for providing me with access to her unpublished war memoir.

My greatest personal thanks go to Professor Christine Hallett for her critical eye, friendship and unswerving belief in my work. None of this would have been possible without her or her support. I am also indebted to both Christine and Professor Jane Schultz, the series editors for *Nursing History and the Humanities*, and Emma Brennan, commissioning editor at Manchester University Press, for their patience, support and valuable advice throughout the writing of the book. I am indebted to the anonymous reviewers for their critical and constructive advice and recommendations. Without their guidance the book would not have done justice to the nursing sisters of the Second World War.

I am most grateful to the editorial and production staff at Manchester University Press for their help, patience and talents in making this book possible. Many of my colleagues in the history of nursing have been most generous with their time, ideas and access to works. My thanks to Carolyn Gibbon and Dr Tommy Dickinson (King's College, London) for reading an early iteration of the proposal for the book and to Professor Peter Nolan for his time and help with the history of mental health nursing. I am most grateful to Dr Cynthia Toman for giving me access to Canadian data, which was unavailable in the UK. My thanks to my colleagues in the Division of Nursing, Midwifery and Social Work at the University of Manchester for supporting me and the history of nursing more widely. In particular, my gratitude goes to Joanne Timpson, colleague and friend. My particular thanks also to my colleague and friend

Dr Nicky Olleveant for reading the manuscript and providing such helpful and constructive advice and suggestions, Professor Karina Lovell, the Director of Research for her support of the history of nursing and both my former and current Heads of School, Professors Karen Luker and Nicky Cullum. Finally thank you to my friends and family and to my husband, James Campbell, for his support, patience and love throughout the process of writing this book.

Abbreviations

BAOR	British Army of the Rhine
BEF	British Expeditionary Force
CCS	Casualty Clearing Station
CMF	Central Mediterranean Force
CO	commanding officer
GH	General Hospital
HMS	His Majesty's Ship
HMHS	His Majesty's Hospital Ship
IWM	Imperial War Museum
IV	intravenous
MEF	Middle East Force
MMM	Museum of Military Medicine (formerly Army Medical Museum)
M.O.	Medical Officer
NHS	National Health Service
PMRAFNS	Princess Mary's Royal Air Force Nursing Service
POW	prisoner of war
QAIMNS/QA	Queen Alexandra's Imperial Military Nursing Service (and the reserve force)
QARANC	Queen Alexandra's Royal Army Nursing Corps
RAF	Royal Air Force
RAMC	Royal Army Medical Corps
RCN	Royal College of Nursing
SOE	Special Operations Executive
TANS	Territorial Army Nursing Service
TNA	The National Archives
VAD	Voluntary Aid Detachment
VD	venereal disease

Introduction

Nursing work and nurses' space in the Second World War: a gendered construction

The Second World War was a new type of war; it was a global, mobile and unpredictable war. It was 'among the most destructive conflicts in human history', in which over forty-six million people perished, often in the most frightening and inhuman conditions.[1] The latter years of the inter-war period witnessed a modernisation of the military technologies that had been used in the First World War. These developments created tanks, submarines and aeroplanes that could transport guns and bombs over vast areas of land and sea far more rapidly than their predecessors could, and with increasingly devastating results. These technologies along with the impulse to use them led the 'commonplace military requirement [to kill] to new depths'.[2]

Improvements in land, sea and airborne transport enabled mass mobilisation of forces into hostile environments such as the deserts of the Middle East and North Africa and the jungles of South-East Asia. Battles that were waged so far from Britain needed men, and even with ever more sophisticated modes of transport it took time to post new soldiers to these far-flung war zones. It was therefore critical to success that men already present in these theatres of war were 'fighting-fit'.[3] The mobility of battles of the Second World War, brought on by 'technological advances in destructive capabilities' necessitated a complete transformation of the techniques needed to manage the injuries and illnesses of war.[4] The frequency of injuries sustained by modern weaponry and the diseases developed in alien places needed a new type of medical service – one that was present near the battle zones and could recover men's bodies quickly to return them to combat. According to medical historian Mark Harrison, the Second World War was the first war in which the Army Medical

Services were understood as critical to the success of the battles; the service was literally 'vital in nursing its men [soldiers] back to health', in order for them to return to fight.[5]

The knowledge that early treatment led to greater success rates meant that for the first time a critical mass of Queen Alexandra's Imperial Military Nursing Service (QA) nurses were posted into these war zones alongside their medical colleagues to provide increasingly complex treatments for combatants.[6] Questions regarding the limits and boundaries of nursing practice meant that the nature of nurses' work has always been contested. Yet on active service overseas the exigencies of war created crisis environments in which these boundaries could be dissolved, enabling more collaborative, less hierarchical work patterns.[7] In *Sisters: Extraordinary True-Life Stories from Nurses in World War Two*, Barbara Mortimer has an image of a nurse and a wounded soldier climbing the gangplank onto the transport ship the *Arundel Castle*. Underneath the image she writes, 'Recovery was hard'.[8] *Negotiating nursing* argues that the QAs, an entirely female force during the Second World War, were critical players in the care of combatants. By renegotiating what counted as nursing work and how nursing work could be performed, nursing sisters were able to support men's physical, emotional and spiritual recovery from illness and injury for the war effort.

The Army Medical Service was not well prepared for war: there was a deficit of over 300 medical officers and in the ranks the shortfall was nearly 3,000.[9] The situation for the QAs was even worse. Santanu Das argues that the operating theatres of the First World War were spaces where the battle between medical science and industrial weaponry was fought by both nurses and doctors, thus nurses had garnered a range of clinical skills.[10] The nursing sisters of the First World War had demonstrated the value of trained, professional nurses to 'contain' the 'trauma' of ill and injured combatants.[11] Yet these skills were lost to military nursing soon after the war ended. The majority of nurses returned to civilian practice or left paid work altogether for what the ideology of the early twentieth century deemed a suitable domestic life, that is, marriage.

Nursing in Britain had been awarded the rights of self-regulation as a registrable profession since 1919, supposedly validating nurses' professional status. However, the caveats to their self-regulation meant it was a 'pyrrhic victory'[12] in which nurses' ability to self-govern were limited by the government.[13] Despite this 'victory', the newly constructed nursing profession was not infiltrated by multitudes of Voluntary Aid Detachment (VAD) nurses, as the trained nurses had feared.[14] Young women had been prepared to nurse as patriotic volunteers during the war, but they had no intention of continuing. According to Janet Watson, of the 120,000 members of the VAD, only 129 used their post-war scholarships to train as a nurse.[15] Thus even those non-professional nurses with war experience were lost to nursing.

The end of the First World War was an anti-climax for most women,[16] who found themselves once more returned to the hearth,[17] although some did make some genuine inroads into public life. The Sex Disqualification (Removal) Act, 1919, theoretically enabled them to engage in civil office. The Representation of the People Act (Equal Franchise) in 1928 enabled 'women to feel that their presence in public life was legitimate'.[18] In reality, although there were some improvements for the women of Britain, most remained liminal to public life and thus ill prepared for the challenges that the next war would bring.

For the nurses of the Second World War, these challenges would be profound. On the eve of the conflict there were only 624 regular nursing officers in the QAs.[19] Hospital matrons had started to recommend certain members of their qualified nursing staff to the QA reservists from about 1933,[20] but the regular force was closed from the declaration of hostilities,[21] something that would have ramifications at the end of the war. The vast majority of nursing sisters who went to war between 1939 and 1945 therefore had no military experience. Few had even been abroad, let alone worked overseas, and many had lived the sheltered lives of young respectable women who moved from the parental home to the hospital Nurses' Home.

The nurses themselves embraced the shift from the physically and psychologically safe spaces of the hospital and Nurses' Home to war.[22] The military medical authorities' appreciation of the sort of hardships that nurses could and should manage was more cautious.[23] Following the declaration of war on 3 September 1939, the female nurses of the British Army were amongst the first contingent of medical services' personnel to enter France. One thousand and three hundred nurses

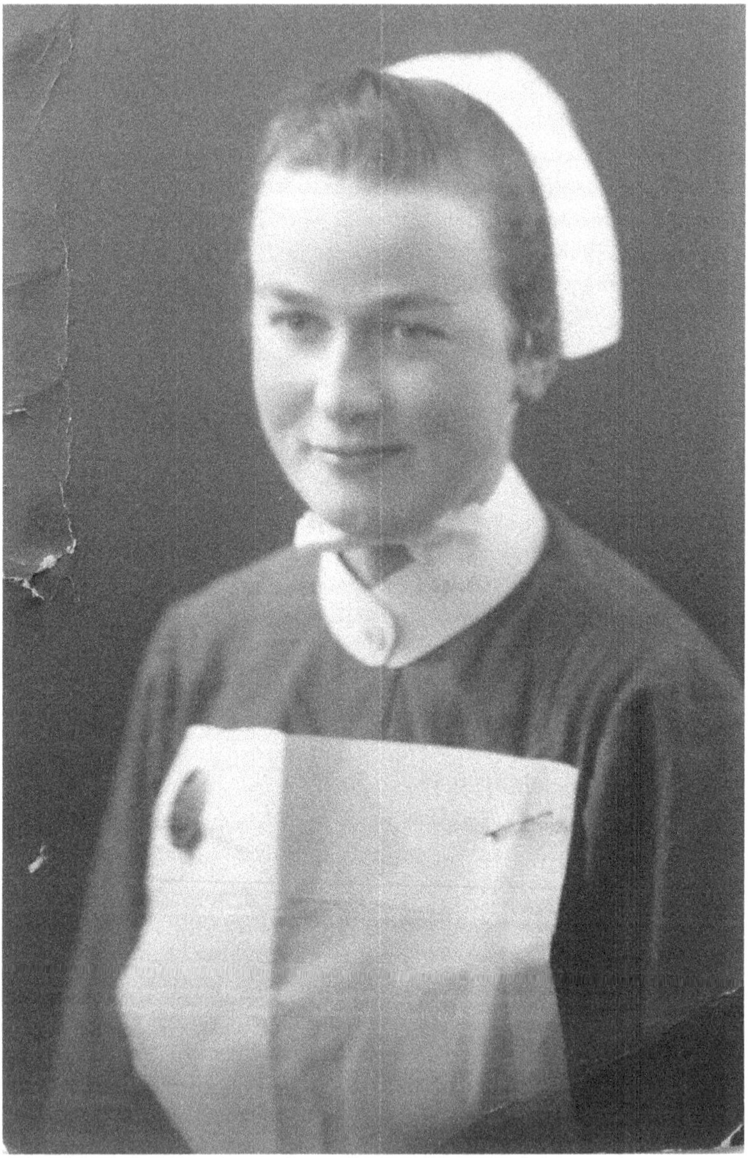

1 Portrait of Nell Jarrett as a student nurse before the war. Here she is shown as the picture of regimented discipline in a starched uniform, closeted into the Nurses' Home.

were evacuated with the British Expeditionary Force in the summer of 1940.[24] Nurses were posted to Africa and the Middle East between 1940 and 1943 and then followed the Army through Italy in 1943 and 1944. Nursing sisters landed in Normandy in June 1944 only days after the Second Front opened and shadowed the troops across Europe and into Germany in 1945. Civilian and Army nurses were present in Asia even before war was declared and were amongst those captured and interned as the Imperial Japanese Army invaded Hong Kong, Singapore and the Philippines in 1941 and 1942. Some internees were not released until September 1945; many died. Finally, nurses were posted to India and Burma to care for soldiers in the South-East Asian war.[25] Thus, despite any anxieties regarding the places to which female nurses could and should be posted, the British Army sent them into and across all war zones.

During the Second World War, the employment of female nurses alongside men of the Royal Army Medical Corps (RAMC) in front-line units engendered if not a transformation then at least a significant revision in the understanding of the roles and work of nursing sisters. The placing of female nurses en masse so close to the front line was a considerable shift in medical policy from previous wars and created a physical space in which to practise that had hitherto eluded them. Furthermore, the acknowledgement of their importance to the war effort that had led to their inclusion in front-line duty raised their confidence. As nurses were posted to ever more hostile places, they started to expect the space to develop their clinical practice and cultivate their position as professional women alongside their male medical colleagues. Space is thus a central concept to the understanding of the position of female nurses in the Second World War. Space denotes not only the physical environment of a war zone or hospital, but also the social space of women. Even into the latter half of the twentieth century, women were understood as occupying the domestic space as help-meet to their husbands and male colleagues.[26] This book examines how the female nurses of the British Army reconstituted women's place in war and nurses' position as the expert at the bedside.

By the last year of the war, what had once been considered inappropriate for female nurses was now expected by senior medical colleagues. Nurses were needed in the most dangerous places to support the healing of men from the most serious and life-threatening conditions. Through their overseas wartime work nursing sisters of the British Armed Forces shifted the understanding of the significance of skilled trained nursing as part of the war effort, what nursing as a women's profession could achieve and attitudes to the participation of women in front-line theatres of war. Yet these women and their work have been largely ignored in histories of the medical services and the wider conflict.

Nursing spaces and nurses' place

Histories of war medicine and rehabilitation provide a critical positioning of nurses in war, although discussions of their work either are entirely absent[27] or tend to be marginalised in the analysis of medical officers and of male patients themselves.[28] In *Medical Services in War*, Francis Albert Eley Crew, the official historian of the Army Medical Services, acknowledged that nursing sisters were vital personnel in the medical services, who raised the standard of care where they were posted: 'The members of the Army Nursing Service would be the first to claim equality with those of the R.A.M.C., in respect to taking risks for the sake of the wounded and the sick. This claim is completely justified by the record of the Q.A.I.M.N.S., during the war.'[29] Nonetheless, he, like others after him, included nurses' work as a side-line to the important role of the medical officers. Both Harrison and Kevin Brown acknowledge the importance of the female nurses of the QAs, although their main focus is on the work of the male medical officers and their care of male soldiers, supported by male orderlies. Harrison's analysis of the nursing sisters is that although there had been some 'friction' between them and the medical officers, they were 'generally admired for their professionalism and technical competence',[30] whereas Brown maintains that female nurses had an important place in base hospitals, caring for ill and injured men under the supervision of medical officers.[31] Therefore, although the professional space of female nurses is portrayed as one of safety and subordination, their work is understood as a vital adjunct to the work of the medical profession.

Where nurses have been considered in more detail, they have frequently been seen as collateral damage and victims to the whims of the medical and military machine, or as heroines to be celebrated for their valour in the face of adversity. Julie Anderson, Emily Mayhew and Liz Byrski demonstrate that although nurses increased the range and complexity of their technical nursing work on the home front, such work did not alter the boundaries of practice.[32] Nurses remained firmly subordinate to the medical profession and their well-being could be sacrificed for the greater good of the men.[33] It is this image of subordination that also alienated nursing from early feminist historians,[34] further hiding their war experiences and work in general.[35] Those celebratory texts that recognise the importance of the nursing sisters' wartime presence,[36] whilst valuable as books that write nurses back into the narrative of the war's medical provision, do not do full service to their essential work.

There are a range of more critical texts about nursing in war in general, but little on the Second World War specifically. Jan Bassett, Mary Sarnecky and Anna Rogers have written highly empirical monographs about Australian, US and New Zealand army nurses, but they cover over 100 years of service.[37] Over recent years there has been a proliferation of work on nursing in the First World War. Most significant of these for the British context are the three monographs by Christine Hallett.[38] These have been an invaluable resource and have been reviewed widely within this book alongside those by Ana Carden-Coyne and Santanu Das.[39] These texts have been further supplemented by works on Dominion nurses by Kirsty Harris and Cynthia Toman.[40] All these texts offer a measure of both continuities and changes between the two world wars.

There are two books that specifically focus on British nursing in the Second World War, but neither analyses the work of nurses. Penny Starns examines the militarisation of nursing during the conflict and the ramifications of that militarisation for nursing in the latter half of the twentieth century.[41] Barbara Mortimer's *Sisters* is an anthology of oral history data taken from the Royal College of Nursing (RCN) archives.[42] This text has proved most valuable for *Negotiating nursing* and is referenced throughout, as it provides additional personal testimony data and some conceptual commentary on the source material. Cynthia Toman's study of Canadian nurses in the Second World War is a particularly important monograph, focusing as it does on the nurses' status as officers and professionals, whilst maintaining their 'respectability as "ladies"' and the contradictions inherent in these multiple identities.[43] There are many similarities in the work and experiences of British and Canadian nurses in the Second World War, but there are also some significant differences. Most notable of these was that Canadian nurses had not as a rule worked in hospitals as registered nurses, but had engaged in private duty nursing. Few Canadian nursing sisters therefore had any significant experience of acute hospital practice post-registration.

Finally, it is worth noting the value of those novels that explore nursing in the Second World War. Ian McEwan's *Atonement*, Michael Ondaatje's *The English Patient* and Monica Dickens' semi-autobiographical *One Pair of Feet*[44] do not form a major part of the analysis in this book, but their focus on the work of nurses supports our understanding of the war and the nurse's place in it. In the introduction to the 1937 edition of *A General Textbook of Nursing*, Evelyn Pearce places the patient at the centre of the nurse's work. According to Pearce, the nurse's only function, and that of the hospital in which she worked, was 'the cure and care of the sick'.[45] By exploring the work of nurses, this book therefore not only provides a unique analysis of nursing sisters in the Second World War – alongside RAMC medical officers and orderlies – but also focuses attention on the military patient as he suffers pain, injury and disease and attempts to recover from the trauma of war to return to battle.

Gendering work

The engagement of female nurses in front-line duty in the Second World War created opportunities for British registered nurses that their peacetime work could not, and that were not present in the hospitals on the home front.[46] Nursing care placed the combatants in a dependent position to women, in direct contrast to the hyper-masculine space of battle from which they had just been removed.[47] In order to care for the more complex cases, female nurses required assistance from male orderlies for hygiene and comfort care, thus placing fit military men in the charge of women. For many men as combatant soldiers and as orderlies, their position as subordinate to women contravened the normal social constructions of gender.[48]

Penny Summerfield and Corinna Peniston-Bird argue that 'the

Second World War was one of the most contradictory periods in British history for the boundary between male and female roles'.[49] According to Juliette Pattinson it was more gender inclusive,[50] as it was the first war into which women were conscripted.[51] Nevertheless, much of the work that women undertook as part of the war effort continued to be gendered.[52] Even when women engaged in dangerous activities, such as espionage, their 'femaleness' was crucial to that work.[53] Some women certainly did move into male work roles such as engineering and welding, but these jobs remained constructed as 'men's jobs'.[54] However, many women simply moved from the kitchen in the home to the kitchen in the factory. Whatever work they did, for the most part it was 'for the duration only', and in war's wake they were returned to the home and hearth.[55]

In many ways the position of female nurses on active service overseas exemplified these contradictions. Nursing was seen as the epitome of female work, yet from 1941 nursing sisters were commissioned officers in the British Army.[56] The highly feminised traditional nurses' uniform was replaced on active service with male battle-dress,[57] ironically in part to preserve female propriety as nurses worked around the stretchers of their male patients.[58] Nursing may have been considered the most female of work, yet nurses were often the only women allowed in the masculine space of a war zone, subverting the 'contract' that men make to protect their womenfolk.[59] Negotiating these sensitive gender boundaries, nurses on active service overseas worked to expand traditional nursing work, developed an autonomy that they had hitherto not known and brokered their place as women in a war zone, 'the one impregnable male bastion'.[60]

Personal testimony and the nurses' war

This book uses a range of personal testimony material, including oral history, diaries, letters and memoirs to examine the work of nurses on active service overseas and their place within the Second World War medical services. Although nursing now, like all other professions, has a written foundation for practice, this is quite a recent phenomenon. Nursing was essentially a profession based on oral rather than written transmission of knowledge.[61] The handover of patient information between shifts on a hospital ward was conducted verbally. Nursing practices were learnt at the bedside, with a more senior nurse both demonstrating and describing the techniques they were using to provide patient care. Arguably, nurses themselves have been much more comfortable speaking of their work and experiences than writing. Given the paucity of written accounts by non-elite nurses, oral history has provided historians of nursing with access to ordinary nurses' working lives, and since the 1990s there has been a proliferation of oral history research on the profession.[62]

The value of oral history over written testimony lies in its 'inter-subjectivity'[63] – that is, the relationship between the interviewer and the narrator that enables the asking of questions and clarification of ideas. This dialogue produces data that provides 'more complex and rounded pictures of the past', and can create an account that fits more specifically with a project's aims.[64] The use of oral history was integral to the research for this book. The fact that I am a nurse supported the development of a narrative that was framed by the interviewees' experiences and my knowledge of nursing and nursing work.[65] This was useful for the research for the book, as it enabled questions to be asked specifically about nursing work, about which non-nurses may struggle to identify and nurses themselves have remained silent.[66] Nurses may have spoken about the professional issues and their training schools, but their work was self-evident. As Elizabeth Bowring, one participant for the study, maintained, 'to care' was 'automatic, it was nursing'.[67]

A key strategy of the project was to give a voice to the few nurses still able to talk about their war, all of whom were over 87 years of age during data collection. In spite of the challenges in accessing women who were approaching or beyond their 90s, over forty retired nurses were located. Most of them were excited about being given the opportunity to talk about their wartime nursing experiences. Unfortunately, there were only four who had been on active service overseas, and not all were able to give an account of their war work. It was therefore necessary to use a number of oral histories that were already in the public domain. The disadvantage of these is that, like written testimony, they do not allow for collaboration between the interviewer and the narrator, thus negating some of the value of the joint participation in an oral history interview.[68] There are also some ethical concerns regarding what Joanna Bornat has called 'revisiting interviews with a different purpose', as it cannot be known if the participants would have consented to their words being used for other projects.[69] Nevertheless, the richness of the interviews has meant that not to include them in the primary source material would be to miss some important perspectives.

All the oral histories identify the war as being a significant point in the nurses' lives, often the most exciting. Being able to discuss their war experiences was an opportunity for catharsis and enabled them to find meaning in their lives, and this was especially so for the majority who after the war entered a traditional life of domesticity and motherhood.[70] Even for those who remained on home soil during the war, the chance to engage in the war effort was seen as amongst the most interesting work of their professional careers. Two participants explicitly voiced their disappointment that the war ended before they had the opportunity for overseas service. Bessie Newton enjoyed nursing soldiers as a student nurse and wanted very much to join the QAs and go overseas, but the war ended before that was possible.[71] Rachel Slater did her tropical diseases training in order to go on active service overseas, but again the war ended and, she said, 'life just took a different course'.[72]

Many research participants were able to remember vividly certain aspects of wartime nursing, especially caring for soldiers in the aftermath of the evacuation from Dunkirk in the late spring of 1940 and the Normandy landings four years later. These memories are framed within what Lynn Abrams refers to as episodic memories – that is, those memories that enable the participant to recall not only an event but also their place in that event.[73] There are potential pitfalls with the memories of Dunkirk and the Normandy landings, which are both overlaid with 70 years of national significance. Dunkirk – so often portrayed as a moment of national pride – was in reality an opportunistic retreat enabled by Hitler's military gaze being focused elsewhere.[74] Nevertheless, this should not be a reason to doubt the memories or their importance for the nurses themselves. Within their 'composed' narratives the nurses also had significant 'flash-bulb' memories of individual patients,[75] suggesting a deeper recollection of details and providing valuable data about the experiences and understandings they had of their work.

In addition to the oral histories, the book makes use of a wide range of personal written testimonies, including private diaries, memoirs and letters.[76] Private correspondence is amongst the most revealing and spontaneous of documentary source material.[77] There is, however, concern that they, like other forms of written evidence, 'lack critical analysis' and are prone to the perceptions, perspectives and agenda of the writer. These personal biases can detract from the promise that they are a lens through which to view true feelings and experiences.[78] Although such material can place the historian close to the event, many documents of this kind are written to entertain, influence or inform.[79] The most sceptical reader of letters and diaries may wonder at the possibility of the authors' blind spots and normal biases or even their capacity for self-deception.[80] In her discussion of nurses' letters from the First World War, Hallett alerts the reader to the difficulties inherent in their interpretation, written as they were for specific audiences.[81] These difficulties are compounded by the lack of replies in the archives and the problems of censorship.

The letters' spontaneity was neutralised by both military censorship and self-censorship. Nurses' letters, as was the case with the correspondence of all military personnel, were monitored to ensure national safety. Given that the 'military actively campaigned to prevent nurses, and indeed all troops, from speaking or writing about their experiences', it is not surprising that letters do not describe the trauma of war, or the nurses' engagement with its victims.[82] Furthermore, most nurses tempered their letters home not only because of official censorship but also to prevent their families from fearing for them; they thus embellished their correspondence with details that made the war sound like 'fun'.[83] There are, however, some notable exceptions. Sister Agnes Morgan's letters home to her mother provide particularly intense descriptions of the horrors of war that both the nurses and the men had to face. It is not clear how Morgan's letters were passed by the censors, or received by her mother, but her stark descriptions of war nursing offer an unusual glimpse into nurses' active service.

Letters are influenced by their audience and require a level of composition that is often based on the anticipated recipient.[84] When that recipient was a family member the descriptions were frequently altered to protect those at home. When the recipient was a nurse herself, the correspondence offers a portrayal of war work that is not present in private correspondence. A key data source of personal testimony for the book was an archive of correspondence, reports and recollections sent by military nurses on active service to the Matron-in-Chief of the British Army, Dame Katharine Jones. This highly valuable resource, because they were written nurse to nurse, contains details of professional practice, the challenges of war nursing and the attitudes of the nurses themselves to their presence in war zones.

The book also makes extensive use of diaries and memoirs, both published and unpublished. Joanne Cooper contends that diaries 'provide us with a map of women's consciousness by describing their daily reality'.[85] Sister Mary Morris's unpublished diary, written almost daily from her student days to the birth of her first child, offers one of the most detailed descriptions of active service life.[86] Morris's reflections on her daily life and work provide a 'template' for her professional development.[87] They suggest courageousness in her nursing practice, in which she was not afraid to develop skills outside the normal remit of nursing or to take risks for her combatant patients. Unlike some diaries that offer limited discussion of nursing work because of the lack of desire to relive the working day, or because nursing work was self-evident, Morris's diary is forthright in its descriptions of Army nursing, the war and her place in it.[88] Reading it, one can sense the unknown as she faces each day without awareness of the next,[89] not knowing whether the Allies would indeed win the war. As it was not written with the intention of publication Morris was able to 'confess' her innermost thoughts[90] without anxieties of impropriety, enabling her to 'relieve feelings aroused by stressful work'.[91]

Sisters Catherine Hutchinson, P.M. Dyer and Catherine Butland's unpublished memoirs are so detailed that they must have been composed from reflections written on active service. However, no original diaries have come to light. All three nurses, like Morris, offer stark descriptions of the mental and physical injury sustained by combatants in war, alongside more humorous and lively anecdotes of active service and social engagements. The memoirs written after the war, both those that were created for the general public and published and also those written for family and friends, notoriously embroider experiences to engender a more palatable war. Like autobiographies, certain memories dominate others, often ignoring the mundane for the more interesting and engaging.[92] They are replete with humour and adventure. Whilst this renders them less empirically reliable,[93] as with oral histories, they demonstrate the composition of women's war experiences as meaningful and valuable, and enabled the writers to craft themselves as 'modern women'.[94]

Chapter outline

Focusing on British Army nurses, this book explores how nurses on active service overseas recovered men within sensitive gender negotiations of what should and could constitute nursing work and where that work could occur. It argues that female nurses in the Second World War suffered similar gendered contradictions to women in general, but also that nursing constituted a special case. The gendered nature of much of nursing work, founded as it was in comfort care and creating homelike spaces, was essentially feminine, having its roots in housekeeping and mothering. On active service overseas, nurses needed to perform this and their more technical roles in hostile places, under fire and with limited human and material resources. These were environments that required skills more commonly associated with educated and professional and therefore, arguably more 'masculine' groups; that is, skills of independent judgement, innovation and critical thinking.[95]

The book moves through an uneven trajectory of the developments of nurses' work, autonomy and the spaces they were allowed to inhabit, to cultivate an understanding of their experiences of caring for combatants. This trajectory should not be understood as one that all nurses followed, nor one that was linear. Rather individual nurses shifted practice as they developed skills and strategies to support their soldier-patients as demanded by the exigencies of war and the challenges that presented in various times and places.

Chapter 1 examines the fundamental nursing work of body and comfort care, feeding work and clinical nursing skills in the face of pain, distress and death. This was care work that all nurses learnt in their hospital training. On active service overseas this work was reformed to provide a more humane nursing service that enabled the healing and recovery of battle-scarred men. However, the development of more personal engagement with their patients was not without difficulty. As the chapter argues, comfort care was overlaid with the threat of sexual frisson, and their patients' pain and death demanded considerable emotional labour from the nurses themselves. Chapter 2 explores challenges to nursing care within the highly mobile war. Many of the difficulties related to the need to create a secure healing space within the harsh environments in which hospitals and casualty clearing stations (CCSs) were situated. The construction of these spaces of safety demanded ingenuity and improvisation on the part of the nursing sisters as they developed wards into homelike places. The importance of the nurses' presence in war zones and the contradictions inherent in their position as women in places of danger are explored in Chapter 3. Military success depended on men sustaining a determination to fight. Persuading men to continue or returning men to combat after illness or injury depended on maintaining their morale. On active service overseas, the use of female nurses in upholding this resolve was integral to the war effort. Yet this posed problems in relation to the sexuality of nurses and raised the spectre of whether they were crucial to the war because they were skilled professionals or because they were women.

War is often understood as a period in which medical advances occur with greater rapidity than in peacetime, and nurses in previous wars had undertaken new and increasingly technological work.[96] In the Second World War nurses once again needed to take on new technologies and scientific work if they were to recover men – work that was conceived as essentially masculine. The rapid development of these technologies meant that often new skills were learnt alongside medical colleagues, and nurses participated in creating new regimes and treatments as members of a team rather than as the medical officers' 'helpmeets'. As Chapter 4 argues, these new skills and technologies became part of the lexicon of nursing work on active service overseas and altered the manner in which nurses and doctors worked to salvage their combatant patients for war. Nevertheless, it was often the autonomy with which they were able to execute the fundamentals of nursing care that provided nursing sisters with a sense of professional and personal pride; autonomy that was lost at war's end. As nurses were demobilised at the end of the war, most simply married. In Chapter 5 the reasons for the decisions not to maintain a professional life are examined, as are the options available to those who could not or would not marry. The testimonies demonstrate a complex interplay of gendered social expectations and reduced professional opportunities which returned experienced military nurses to the domestic setting and precluded them from taking their highly developed nursing skills into the new National Health Service (NHS). Despite these professional disappointments, the nurses' testimonies bear witness to the impact that their overseas war service had on the understanding of what nursing could achieve. *Negotiating nursing* argues that in multiple ways, through fundamental care, the creation of homelike spaces, nurses' presence as women in a war zone and the development of scientific modes of practice, the nursing sisters of the British Army recovered combatant patients from the battlefield and for the war.

Notes

1 Martin Gilbert, *The Second World War: A Complete History* (London: Phoenix, 2009), 1.

2 Joanna Bourke, *The Second World War: A People's History* (Oxford: Oxford University Press, 2001), 1.

3 Kevin Brown, *Fighting Fit: Health, Medicine and War in the Twentieth Century* (Stroud: The History Press, 2008).

4 Susan Gubar, '"This is my rifle, this is my gun": World War II and the blitz on women', in Margaret Randolph Higonnet, Jane Jenson, Sonya Michel and Margaret Collins Weitz (eds), *Behind the Lines: Gender and the Two World Wars* (New Haven, CT: Yale University Press, 1987), 230.

5 Mark Harrison, *Medicine and Victory: British Military Medicine in the Second World War* (Oxford: Oxford University Press, 2004), 2.

6 Julie Anderson, *War, Disability and Rehabilitation in Britain: 'Soul of a Nation'* (Manchester: Manchester University Press, 2011), 76.

7 Jane Brooks and Christine E. Hallett, 'Introduction: The practice of nursing and the exigencies of war', in Jane Brooks and Christine E. Hallett (eds), *One Hundred Years of Wartime Nursing Practices, 1854–1953* (Manchester: Manchester University Press, 2015), 1.

8 Barbara Mortimer, *Sisters: Extraordinary True-Life Stories from Nurses in World War Two* (London: Hutchinson, 2012), 180.

9 Harrison, *Medicine and Victory*, 30. F.A.E. Crew argued that 'The fact that so small a body should have been capable of providing so firm a foundation for the superstructure it was subsequently called upon to maintain, merits some description of its nature and development'. F.A.E. Crew, *The Army Medical Services: Volume I: Administration* (London: HMSO, 1953), 3.

10 Santanu Das, *Touch and Intimacy in First World War Literature* (Cambridge: Cambridge University Press, 2005).

11 Christine E. Hallett, *Containing Trauma: Nursing Work in the First World War* (Manchester: Manchester University Press, 2009). See also Christine E. Hallett, *Veiled Warriors: Allied Nurses of the First World War* (Oxford: Oxford University Press, 2014); Christine E. Hallett, '"This fiendish mode of warfare": Nursing the victims of gas poisoning in the First World War', in Jane Brooks and Christine E. Hallett (eds), *One Hundred Years of Wartime Nursing Practices, 1854–1953* (Manchester: Manchester University Press, 2015); Christine E. Hallett, *Nurse Writers of the Great War* (Manchester: Manchester University Press, 2016). For a wider review of the work of nursing sisters from Dominion countries, see also Cynthia Toman, *Sister Soldiers of the Great War: The Nurses of the Canadian Army Medical Corps* (Vancouver: University of British Columbia Press, 2016); Kirsty Harris, '"Health, healing and harmony": Invalid cookery and feeding by Australian nurses in the Middle East in the First World War', in Jane Brooks and Christine E. Hallett (eds), *One Hundred Years of Wartime Nursing Practices, 1854–1953* (Manchester: Manchester University Press, 2015); Kirsty Harris, *More than Bombs and Bandages: Australian Army Nurses at Work in World War I* (Newport: Big Sky Publishing, 2011); Ruth Rae, *Scarlet Poppies: The Army Experience of Australian Nurses during World War I* (Burwood: College of Nursing, 2004).

12 Monica Baly, *Nursing and Social Change* (London: Routledge, 1995), 154.

13 Anne Marie Rafferty, *The Politics of Nursing Knowledge* (London: Routledge, 1996), 93; Robert Dingwall, Anne Marie Rafferty and Charles Webster, *An Introduction to the Social History of Nursing* (London: Routledge, 1988), 88.

14 Rafferty, *The Politics of Nursing Knowledge*, 78.

15 Janet S. Watson, 'Wars in the wards: The social construction of medical work in First World War Britain', *Journal of British Studies* 41, 4 (2002): 510. See also Janet S.K. Watson, 'Khaki girls, VADs, and Tommy's sister: Gender and class in First World War Britain', *The International History Review* 19, 1 (1997): 32–50; Janet S.K. Watson, *Fighting Different Wars: Experience, Memory, and the First World War in Britain* (Cambridge: Cambridge University Press, 2007).

16 Anne Summers, *Angels and Citizens: British Women as Military Nurses, 1854–1914* (Newbury: Threshold Press, 2000), 249.

17 Adrian Bingham, '"An era of domesticity": Histories of women and gender in interwar Britain', *Cultural and Social History* 1 (2004): 227.

18 Pat Thane, 'What difference did the vote make? Women in public and private life in Britain since 1918', *Historical Research* 76, 192 (2003): 285. For detailed discussions regarding the changes to women's lives following the franchise, see, for example, Maria DiCenzo, '"Our freedom and its results": Measuring progress in the aftermath of suffrage', *Women's History Review* 23, 3 (2014): 421–40; Barbara Caine, *English Feminism, 1780–1980* (Oxford: Oxford University Press, 2001); Caitriona Beaumont, 'Citizens not feminists: The boundary negotiated between citizenship and feminism by mainstream

women's organisations in England, 1928–39', *Women's History Review* 9, 2 (2000): 411–29; Caitriona Beaumont, 'The women's movement, politics and citizenship, 1918–1950s', in Ina Zweiniger-Bargielowska (ed.), *Women in Twentieth-Century Britain* (Harlow: Pearson Education, 2001).

19 Katharine H. Jones, 'Introduction', in Ada Harrison (ed.), *Grey and Scarlet: Letters From the War Areas by Army Sisters on Active Service* (London: Hodder and Stoughton, 1944), 8. Reprinted in *The British Journal of Nursing* (March 1944): 29.

20 Nicola Tyrer, *Sisters in Arms: British Army Nurses Tell their Story* (London: Phoenix, 2008), 17.

21 Penny Starns, *Nurses at War: Women on the Frontline, 1939–45* (Stroud: Sutton Publishing, 2000), 13.

22 According to the retired Second World War nurses interviewed for 'Frontline Females' on BBC Radio 4, some felt that nurses could be forgiven for seeing war as a golden opportunity not only to serve but to advance themselves professionally, 'so when war was declared, there was a stampede to join up'. The more prosaic amongst them maintained, 'nurses needed a job and this offered an excellent opportunity'. 'Frontline Females', BBC Radio 4, 11 April 1998: British Library Sound Archive H9872/2. In this programme Claire Rayner discussed their wartime nursing experiences with: Monica Baly, Mary Bates, Glenys Branson, Constance Collingwood, Gertrude Cooper, Ursula Dowling, Brenda Fuller, Anne Gallimore, Monica Goulding, Daphne Ingram, Anita Kelly, Margaret Kneebone, Sylvia Mayo, Kay McCormack, Anne Moat, Phyllis Thoms and Margot Turner. Individual nurses were not introduced as they spoke, so it is not possible to determine who held which views.

23 F.A.E. Crew suggested that nursing sisters were needed for the Middle East, but that they should be volunteers who did not mind the hardships inherent in the campaign. In this Crew appears to be suggesting that women were different to men and should be treated more carefully. F.A.E. Crew, *The Army Medical Services: Volume II: Campaigns: Hong Kong, Malaya, Iceland and the Faroes, Libya, 1942–1943, North West Africa* (London: HMSO, 1957), 393.

24 Katharine H. Jones, 'Introduction', in Ada Harrison (ed.), *Grey and Scarlet: Letters From the War Areas by Army Sisters on Active Service* (London: Hodder and Stoughton, 1944), 10.

25 There are a vast number of texts on the Second World War and its battles. For a comprehensive and highly detailed account, see Gilbert, *The Second World War*. For a more abbreviated text, see Bourke, *The Second World War*.

26 The idea that women occupy a 'separate sphere' to men is the subject of many texts on women's history. For a detailed and comprehensive analysis, see, for example, Amanda Vickery, 'Historiographical review: Golden age to separate spheres? A review of the categories and chronology of English women's history', *The Historical Journal* 36, 2 (1993): 383–414.

27 Emma Newlands, *Civilians into Soldiers: War, the Body and British Army Recruits, 1939–45* (Manchester: Manchester University Press, 2014).

28 In his article on the growth of literature on medicine and war, Mark Harrison states that 'there are signs that health and medicine are at last moving centre-stage in British military historiography', although he does not mention nursing per se. Mark Harrison, 'The medicalization of war – the militarization of medicine', *The Society for the Social History of Medicine* 9, 2 (1996): 269.

29 F.A.E. Crew, 'The Army Nursing Service', in Arthur Salusbury MacNalty and W. Frankin Mellor (eds), *Medical Services in War: The Principal Medical Lessons of the Second World War* (London: HMSO), 80. Crew was attached to the War Office during the Second World War, and later held the Chair in Social and Preventative Medicine at the University of Edinburgh.

30 Harrison, *Medicine and Victory*, 32

31 Brown, *Fighting Fit.*

32 Emily Mayhew, *The Reconstruction of Warriors: Archibald McIndoe, The Royal Air Force and the Guinea Pig Club* (Barnsley: Greenhill Books, 2010); Anderson, *War, Disability and Rehabilitation in Britain*; Liz Byrski, 'Emotional labour as war work: Women up close and personal with McIndoe's Guinea Pigs', *Women's History Review* 21, 3 (2012): 341–61.

33 Anderson, *War, Disability and Rehabilitation in Britain*; Byrski, 'Emotional labour as war work'.

34 June Purvis, 'Using primary sources when researching women's history from a feminist perspective', *Women's History Review* 1, 2 (1992): 274. Martha Vicinus' 1985 monograph, *Independent Women: Work and Community for Single Women, 1850–1920*, is a case in point. Whilst her explorations of women's religious and academic communities are largely positive, her portrayal of the nursing profession and its members is highly critical. Martha Vicinus, *Independent Women* (London: Virago, 1985).

35 For example, Braybon and Summerfield do consider nursing in *Out of the Cage*, but only as an illustration of a 'women's profession'. Where they examine the war work of nurses, the reference to professional nurses is fleeting (p. 44), whereas the only detailed episode of war nursing work uses a quotation from a VAD nurse (p. 65). Gail Braybon and Penny Summerfield, *Out of the Cage: Women's Experiences in Two World Wars* (London: Pandora, 1987).

36 Ian Hay, *One Hundred Years of Army Nursing: The Story of the British Army Nursing Services from the Time of Florence Nightingale to the Present Day* (London: Cassell, 1953); Juliet Piggott, *Queen Alexandra's Royal Army Nursing Corps* (London: Leo Cooper, 1975); Brenda McBryde, *Quiet Heroines: Nurses of the Second World War* (London: Chatto and Windus, 1985); Eric Taylor, *Front-Line Nurse: British Nurses in World War II* (London: Robert Hale, 1997); Eric Taylor, *Wartime Nurse: One Hundred Years from the Crimea to Korea, 1854–1954* (London: Robert Hale, 2001); Tyrer, *Sisters in Arms.*

37 Jan Bassett, *Guns and Brooches: Australian Army Nursing from the Boer War to the Gulf War* (Oxford: Oxford University Press, 1992); Mary Sarnecky, *A History of the US Army Nurse Corps* (Philadelphia, PA: University of Pennsylvania Press, 1999); Anna Rogers, *While You're Away: New Zealand Nurses at War, 1899–1948* (Auckland: Auckland University Press, 2003).

38 Hallett, *Containing Trauma*; Hallett, *Veiled Warriors*; Hallett, *Nurse Writers.*

39 Ana Carden-Coyne, *The Politics of Wounds: Military Patients and Medical Power in the First World War* (Oxford: Oxford University Press, 2014); Das, *Touch and Intimacy.*

40 Harris, *More than Bombs and Bandages*; Toman, *Sister Soldiers.*

41 Starns, *Nurses at War.*

42 Barbara Mortimer, *Sisters: Extraordinary True-Life Stories from Nurses in World War Two* (London: Hutchinson, 2012).

43 Cynthia Toman, *An Officer and a Lady: Canadian Military Nursing and the Second World War* (Vancouver: University of British Columbia Press, 2007), 93.

44 Michael Ondaatje, *The English Patient* (London: Bloomsbury, 1992); Ian McEwan, *Atonement* (London: Vintage Books, 2002); Monica Dickens, *Chronicle of a Working Life*: *One Pair of* Feet (Stroud: Sutton Publishing, 2004).

45 Evelyn Pearce, *A General Textbook of Nursing: A Comprehensive Guide to the Final State Examinations* (London: Faber and Faber, 1937), 1.

46 Mayhew, *The Reconstruction of Warriors*; Anderson, *War, Disability and Rehabilitation in Britain.*

47 Gubar, '"This is my rifle, this is my gun"; Harrison, *Medicine and Victory*; Mayhew, *The Reconstruction of Warriors*; Anderson, *War, Disability and Rehabilitation in Britain.*

48 The difficulties that men experienced with these gender reconfigurations were exacerbated by attitudes to the loss of manliness to both injury and illness and also the position of men in non-combatant roles. Anderson, *War, Disability and Rehabilitation in Britain*; Carden-Coyne, *The Politics of Wounds*; Lucy Noakes, '"Serve to save": Gender, citizenship and Civil Defence in Britain, 1937–41', *Journal of Contemporary History* 47, 4 (2012): 737.

49 Penny Summerfield and Corinna Peniston-Bird, 'Women in the firing-line: The Home Guard and the defence of gender boundaries in Britain in the Second World War', *Women's History Review* 9, 2 (2000): 232.

50 Juliette Pattinson, *Behind Enemy Lines: Gender, Passing and the Special Operations Executive in the Second World War* (Manchester: Manchester University Press, 2007), 13.

51 Sonya O. Rose, *Which People's War? National Identity and Citizenship in Britain, 1939–1945* (Oxford: Oxford University Press, 2003).

52 Penny Summerfield, 'Women and war in the twentieth century', in June

Purvis (ed.), *Women's History: Britain, 1850–1945* (London: UCL Press, 1995); Penny Summerfield, *Reconstructing Women's Wartime Lives: Discourse and Subjectivity in Oral Histories of the Second World War* (Manchester: Manchester University Press, 1998).

53 Pattinson, *Behind Enemy Lines.*

54 Susan R. Grayzel, '"Fighting for the idea of home life": *Mrs Miniver* and Anglo-American representations of domestic morale', in Philippa Levine and Susan R. Grayzel (eds), *Gender, Labour, War and Empire* (London: Palgrave Macmillan, 2009).

55 Gail Braybon and Penny Summerfield, *Out of the Cage: Women's Experiences in Two World Wars* (London: Pandora, 1987); Deborah Montgomerie, 'Reassessing Rosie: World War II, New Zealand women and the iconography of femininity', *Gender and History* 8, 1 (1996): 108–32; Phil Goodman, '"Patriotic femininity": Women's morals and men's morale during the Second World War', *Gender and History* 10, 2 (1998): 278–93; Summerfield, *Reconstructing Women's Wartime Lives*; Sheila Rowbotham, *A Century of Women: A History of Women in Britain and the United States* (London: Penguin, 1999).

56 Katharine Jones, 'QAIMNS professional and military status', *Nursing Times* (27 January 1945): 60.

57 Katharine Jones, 'On active service with the Army', *Nursing Times* (25 September 1943): 719.

58 Geraldine Edge and Mary E. Johnstone, *Ships of Youth: The Experiences of Two Army Nursing Sisters on Board the Hospital Carrier Leinster* (London: Hodder and Stoughton, 1945), 18.

59 Christina Twomey, 'Australian nurse POWs: Gender, war and captivity', *Australian Historical Studies* 36, 124 (2004): 255–74.

60 John Laffin, *Women in Battle* (London: Abelard Schuman, 1967), 11.

61 Narelle Biedermann, 'The voices of days gone by: Advocating the use of oral history in nursing', *Nursing Inquiry* 8 (2001): 61.

62 Oral history is acknowledged by its protagonists as being instrumental in enabling the voice of the ordinary person to be heard. It is therefore highly valuable in researching working-class history, women's history and, in this instance, non-elite nurses. Lynn Abrams, *Oral History Theory* (London: Routledge, 2010), 27. It is not the intention here to discuss the variety of oral history research, but see, for example, Abrams, *Oral History Theory*; Paul Thompson, *The Voice of the Past: Oral History* (Oxford: Oxford University Press, 2000); Robert Perks and Alastair Thomson, *The Oral History Reader* (London: Routledge, 1998); Joan Sangster, '"Telling our stories": Feminist debates and the use of oral history', *Women's History Review* 3, 1 (1994): 5–28. For a discussion on methodological issues of oral history in nursing history, see Geertje Boschma, Erica Roberts, Ranjit Dhari, Gilda Mahabir, Susan Walter and Catherine Haney, '"Nobody ever asked me about my career": Public health nurses' oral histories preserved', *The Bulletin of the*

UK Association for the History of Nursing 4 (2015): 43–51; Geertje Boschma, Margaret Scaia, Nerrisa Bonifacio and Erica Roberts, 'Oral history research', in Sandra B. Lewenson and Eleanor Krohn Herrmann (eds), *Capturing Nursing History: A Guide to Historical Methods in Research* (New York: Springer, 2008); Olga M. Church and M.L. Johnson, 'Worth remembering: The process and products of oral history', *International History of Nursing Journal* 1, 1 (1995): 23–4.

63 According to Lynn Abrams this intersubjectivity is based on a 'three-way dialogue' that exists during the interview. First, the dialogue the participant has with themselves, second, the conversation between the participant and the interviewer and third, between the interviewer and their 'cultural discourses'. Abrams, *Oral History Theory*, 59. In written personal testimonies or in oral histories that are revisited by another researcher for a different reason, that central aspect of the dialogue is missing, thus the dialogue between the past and present is broken in away that does not happen in the oral history interview.

64 Graham J. Thurgood, 'Nurses' voices from the archives', *Journal of the Society of Archivists* 31, 2 (2010): 140.

65 Tommy Dickinson, *'Curing Queers': Mental Nurses and their Patients, 1935–74* (Manchester: Manchester University Press, 2015), 10.

66 David Justham, '"Those maggots – they did a wonderful job": The nurses' role in wound management in civilian hospitals during the Second World War', in Jane Brooks and Christine E. Hallett (eds), *One Hundred Years of Nursing Wartime Practices, 1854–1953* (Manchester: Manchester University Press, 2015), 190.

67 Elizabeth Bowring, oral history interview via telephone by Jane Brooks, 31 July 2012.

68 Sherna Berger Gluck and Daphne Patai, 'Introduction', in Sherna Berger Gluck and Daphne Patai (eds), *Women's Words: The Feminist Practice of Oral History* (London: Routledge, 1991), 2.

69 Joanna Bornat, 'A second take: Revisiting interviews with a different purpose', *Oral History* 31, 1 (2003): 47–53.

70 Mahua Sarkar, 'Between craft and method: Meaning and inter-subjectivity in oral history analysis', *Journal of Historical Sociology* 25, 4 (2012): 578–600; Lynn Abrams, 'Liberating the female self: Epiphanies, conflict and coherence in the life stories of post-war British women', *Social History* 39, 1 (2014): 14–35.

71 Bessie Newton, oral history interview at her home in Yorkshire by Jane Brooks, 21 April 2012.

72 Rachel Slater, oral history interview in the South of England by Jane Brooks, 20 October 2011.

73 Abrams, *Oral History Theory*, 83.

74 Harrison, *Medicine and Victory*, 52.

75 Penny Summerfield, 'Culture and composure: Creating narratives of the gendered self in oral history interviews', *Cultural and Social History* 1 (2004): 66. For a detailed analysis of 'composure' in oral history, see also Summerfield, *Reconstructing Women's Wartime Lives.*

76 I have been fortunate to receive a number of unpublished diaries, journals and essays of nurses from their family members, and I am most grateful for these accounts. Although the provenance of material that has not been validated by an archivist cannot be assured, several were handwritten, in clearly old notebooks and diaries. Those that were typed, such as the unpublished memoir from Jessie Wilson, came with a covering letter by her nephew, with details of Wilson's life and death.

77 John Tosh, *The Pursuit of History* (London: Longman Publishing, 2002), 70; Olga Kenyon, *800 Years of Women's Letters* (Stroud: Alan Sutton Publishing, 1992), vii.

78 Sandra B. Lewenson, 'Doing historical research', in Sandra B. Lewenson and Eleanor Krohn Herrmann (eds), *Capturing Nursing History: A Guide to Historical Methods in Research* (New York: Springer, 2008), 34.

79 Tosh, *The Pursuit of History*, 62.

80 Anthony Brundage, *Going to the Sources: A Guide to Historical Research and Writing* (Hoboken, NJ: Wiley Blackwell, 2017), 17.

81 Hallett, *Containing Trauma*, 11.

82 Toman, *An Officer and a Lady*, 72.

83 Toman, *An Officer and a Lady*, 73.

84 Joanne E. Cooper, 'Shaping meaning: Women's diaries, journals and letters – the old and the new', *Women's Studies International Forum* 10, 1 (1987): 96.

85 Cooper, 'Shaping meaning', 95.

86 Since commencing the book this diary has been published in an abridged form. Where the original diary and the published one correspond, both references are provided. Mary Morris, *A Very Private Diary: A Nurse in Wartime*, ed. Carol Acton (London: Weidenfeld and Nicolson, 2014).

87 Alison Twells, '"Went into raptures": Reading emotion in the ordinary wartime diary, 1941–1946', *Women's History Review* 25, 1 (2016): 144.

88 Carol Acton, '"Stepping into history": Reading the Second World War through Irish women's diaries', *Irish Studies Review* 18, 1 (2010): 43.

89 Cooper, 'Shaping meaning', 99.

90 Tosh, *The Pursuit of History*, 72. Joanne Cooper also identifies with this semi-confessional, almost prayer aspect of the daily diary. Cooper, 'Shaping meaning', 95.

91 Christine E. Hallett, 'The personal writings of First World War nurses: A study of the interplay of authorial intention and scholarly interpretation', *Nursing Inquiry* 14, 4 (2007): 322.

92 Lucy Noakes, *War and the British: Gender, Memory and National Identity* (London: I.B. Tauris, 1998), 80–1.

93 Hallett, *Containing Trauma*, 12.
94 Abrams, 'Liberating the female self', 19.
95 Michael Traynor, Maggie Boland and Niels Buus, 'Autonomy, evidence and intuition: Nurses and decision-making', *Journal of Advanced Nursing* 66, 7 (2010): 1584–91; Sylvia Walby and June Greenwell, *Medicine and Nursing: Professions in a Changing Health Service* (London: Sage, 1994).
96 Roger Cooter and Steve Sturdy, 'Of war, medicine and modernity', in Roger Cooter, Mark Harrison and Steve Sturdy (eds), *Medicine and Modern Warfare* (Amsterdam: Rodopi, 1998); Hallett, *Containing Trauma*; Jane Brooks and Christine E. Hallett (eds), *One Hundred Years of Nursing Wartime Practices, 1854–1953* (Manchester: Manchester University Press, 2015).

1

Salvaging soldiers, comforting men

On 2 September 1939, the eve of the Second World War, the *Nursing Mirror* declared that a nurse 'is not brought up to expect ease and comfort, but rather to learn to create ease and comfort for others'.[1] This chapter examines the role of military nurses in war zones across the globe in providing this 'ease and comfort' for their combatant patients, and doing so in increasingly confident and humanitarian modes. Preparations began for the mobilisation of the Queen Alexandra's Imperial Military Nursing Service (QAs), their Reserve and the Territorial Army Nursing Service (TANS)[2] from the mid-1930s as war seemed ever more inevitable. Orders then commenced on 1 September 1939, when at one o'clock the War Office in London contacted the QA Matron-in-Chief: 'Mobilisation orders received. Complete mobilisation of QAIMNS + QAIMNS Res came into effect. Matron-in-Chief QAIMNS to move her office from 3 Spring Gardens to 3 Thames House on 2.9.39.'[3] The first members of the QAs and their Reserve left for France on 10 September. By 25 September, 570 nurses had embarked for France. Nursing sisters of the British Army were eventually posted to all war zones of the Second World War to care for combatants.

The chapter maps the nursing practices on active service overseas that recovered men, including body care, feeding work, the management of pain and support for the dying. These four areas of nursing practice are commonly associated with nursing work, yet, in war zones, they demanded complex gendered brokery. The intimacy of body care, the moment when the single young female nurse meets the young male patient, required skilful negotiations in order to alleviate the spectre of unrestrained sexuality.[4] Feeding work was quintessentially part of women's domestic role, but during the Second World War it took on political import as women fed the nation on rations and saved Britain from waste. Military nurses demonstrated that they too had the skills and ingenuity to scavenge, prepare and administer nutritious food to recover men for battle. The care of pain was crucial to patient recovery and yet, in the masculine space of war, the combatant was often reluctant to admit to it. Thus nurses needed to use skilful techniques of assessment and management in the face of the soldier's stoicism to provide him with adequate pain relief. As part of the formation of skills to manage their combatant patients in war zones overseas, nurses developed the artistry of their practice from task orientation to a humanitarian service that healed men physically, socially and emotionally, in order to prepare them for return to the battlefield, or support them in death.[5]

As men were laid waste across the globe by the destructive forces of modern weaponry, military nurses were posted to all war zones in unprecedented numbers, and contrary to gendered expectations. Cynthia Toman argues in regard to the Canadian military nursing service that 'It was gender, not nurses' abilities that constrained their work'.[6] But gender also was the key to their war work. Combatants in dangerous war zones had historically been cared for by male orderlies. By the Second World War, medical military authorities were armed with the knowledge that successful medical outcomes were more likely with earlier treatment. In order to provide prompt, expert care, trained nurses were needed close to the fighting. Despite the fact that some of the orderlies were themselves registered nurses, the decision was taken to post female nurses to front-line duty.[7] Although as Crew wrote, 'male and female nurses can be completely equal in response to professional knowledge and skill', he continued that the chief and most important difference was their gender. The ill or injured combatant 'is a child-like creature, often dependent and insecure, who sees in the female nurse a mother-figure, tender and compassionate'.[8] Nevertheless, nurses' training had not necessarily prepared them for the tender ministrations needed to salvage their soldier-patients.

Transforming nursing care

The testimonies of nurses acknowledged that their regimented and highly disciplined training was in many ways 'dehumanising'. For those who qualified as registered nurses and went on active service overseas, there was also an appreciation that this training toughened them and thus enabled them to manage the challenges of war nursing. The long hours, hard work and sometimes overly harsh regimes prepared them for war and its human tragedy as the skills they learnt as student nurses became embedded in their 'nursing-selves'. Writing in her diary after arriving in Normandy shortly after D-Day, Sister Ann Radloff stated, 'This was the moment for which I had prepared for four long years, and during which, as well as fun and friendship, I had suffered depersonalisation, despair, discipline and desolation.'[9] Sister Brenda McBryde landed in Normandy with the 81 British General Hospital also in June 1944. In her memoir she described 'the trauma' of her first day in the resuscitation department:

> Everything I had learned during four hard years of training suddenly made sense. My hands had a sure and certain skill and my brain was unflustered as I replaced dressings over gaping wounds, gave injections of morphia and the new wonder drug, penicillin, charted blood pressures. I began to see, for the first time, that the disciplines of the training school were a necessary part of the whole. That tent, full of men, whose clammy bodies overpowered me with the nauseous sweet smell of shock were my fulfilment, since they could no longer help themselves.[10]

The regimented training of nurses in British hospitals in the 1930s and early 1940s thus enabled those nurses who went on active service overseas to perform bodily care and clinical nursing work, despite the alien environments in which they found themselves. In a letter to her mother from active service in Italy, Sister Agnes Morgan described her elation at being able to engage in 'real war-nursing ... bandaging, giving injections, washing, lifting, dressing – no red tape, no beds to make, no rules or regulations to observe', and with no supervision.[11] Here she offered a list of the same work that all nurses would have engaged in on wards in civilian hospitals in Britain, work that was the backbone of their duties. The lack of supervision and the new delights at a more autonomous mode of practice were novel experiences. Just like Hana in *The English Patient* who muses that 'She would not be ordered again',[12] it was this autonomy that Morgan, like many of her Army nursing colleagues, welcomed as part of active service. Yet two years earlier, in a letter from Egypt, she had acknowledged the need to care not only for the bodies of the men, but also for their humanity.

> By night they came on convoys broken and maimed and what could we do but give them everything we had in the way of nursing skill and bodily comforts, and by day they came in walking (like the Welchmen from Benghazi), often maimed in mind, but only exhausted in body, and now what comforts had we for these? What wise council, what heroic words would sooth a haunted mind?[13]

Nurses' training had clearly prepared them to care of the 'broken and maimed' bodies of men. Morgan was not so sure how it prepared them for the emotional care required to recover men from the physical and psychological trauma of war and to see the patient as a person.[14] As Radloff argued, her posting to active service overseas was the 'beginning of involvement in such courage, patience, tragedy, torment and laughter that was to transform us all into different people'.[15]

Caring for bodies, recovering men

Sister Angela Bolton maintained that her nursing routines in India during the Second World War had been very similar to those in England before the war. The day started with sisters' and doctors' rounds, dressings, medicines and patients' meals.[16] Despite body care being the mainstay of nursing work, she does not list it in her daily duties. Over the past century areas of nursing practice have been transformed and transferred to other professions. Massage became the province of physiotherapists, nutrition the work of dieticians and X-rays that of radiographers.[17] Hygiene and elimination care stayed with nursing, yet are the least discussed areas of nursing practice in the personal testimonies, as the reference to Bolton's daily work above suggests. There are arguably three reasons for the hidden nature of this work, given censorship rules and nurses' self-censorship. One reason is body care's self-evidence as nursing work. Second, body and hygiene care are inextricably associated with dirt; third are concerns that the potential sexual undertones in the encounter between the female nurse and her male combatant patient could not easily be nullified.[18]

War should be a masculine space,[19] and yet the status of being a patient is bound in dependency.[20] Dwelling on the weakness of the ill or injured soldier may have provided a safer narrative for the nursing sisters, but it did not render body care benign. Joanna Bourke argues that for those disabled from birth, a level of passivity surrounds their being. The injured soldier was, however, both mutilator and mutilated; he was a man whose passivity is contingent: 'He was the fit man, the potent man *rendered* impotent.'[21] The mobility of the Second World War meant that female nurses were often far away from the supervision of older nurses. Their work and relative autonomy carried with them dangers of impropriety and sexual frisson.[22] The patriotic duty of female nurses may have been to salvage men for the battlefield or to return them to their loved ones at home, but such unfettered closeness could carry with it public and private fears of sexual freedoms and a disruption of accepted social relations.[23]

Discussions on the difficulties that war created for anticipated female propriety fill texts on women's wartime work. According to Sonya O. Rose, with the advent of the war, concern over the behaviour of young women was brought into stark relief.[24] Even for those women on home soil there was a great deal of suspicion about women in uniform,[25] the wearing of which suggested gender bending[26] and women's active participation in the conflict.[27] The shifting of nurses' space from the hospital in Britain to the ward in a war zone transformed her from feminine home-maker to war worker. As Cynthia Enloe argues, military nursing sat on an 'ideological knife-edge',[28] exacerbated by nurses' proximity to naked male patients.

The care of the male body by young, single women thus placed nurses in a liminal place between the accepted face of femininity and the ambiguities of heterosexual touch.[29] The nurses themselves were clearly aware of this, although they rarely articulated their concerns explicitly. When Sister Mary Morris was posted with the 101 British General Hospital to Louvain in Belgium, the building that was destined to be their hospital was a converted convent of closed nuns. Morris stated that the nuns were 'delighted to have us', despite the fact that 'men have not been part of their lives'.[30] Later in her diary, on 16 October 1944, Morris admitted, 'The nuns here are an enormous help to me, particularly Marie Anselma. It must be extremely difficult for her to cope with the nursing duties here – some of which are very intimate and difficult.'[31] In her semi-autobiographical book based on her war experiences, Sister Pamela Bright admitted to the confusion and embarrassment felt by her and her colleagues when 'our patients showed a frank consciousness of sex'.[32] Arguably, it is highly significant that this blunt admission occurs in a text that is only 'based' on her war experiences and not taken from a diary or letters. Whilst the full range of testimonies used in this book contains comprehensive descriptions of nursing work, detailed discussions of bodily care are often notable by their absence, and the two quotes above are the only places where the spectre of sex is recognised.

The work of the nurse in caring for people's bodily functions is such a truism that it neither needs to be nor should be discussed.[33] Furthermore, given nurses' privileged status as white female officers, they may not have wished to acknowledge body work, even to themselves. As nursing reform became embedded in the hospital services of nineteenth-century Britain, the engagement with patient hygiene meant that in the embodiment of the single, female nurse, 'women's purity and impurity were expressed at once morally and physically'.[34] Nurses were not only agents of reform, but also potentially suspect. In order to maintain a level of propriety they were advised to be quiet about the more unpleasant aspects of their work.[35] For, as Leonore Davidoff argued, those who engaged in 'dirty work' not only became defiled by the association with dirt, but also could themselves become the defiler.[36] In the nineteenth and early twentieth centuries the body work of nurses was imbued with a 'nursing-as-Christian-practice discourse' in order to circumvent impropriety and promote an ideology of middle-class morality.[37] Nurses needed to be symbols of Christian chastity in order to have the respect of male patients whilst they provided 'intimate ministrations'.[38] Florence Nightingale herself demanded that women who entered nursing should acknowledge that the work 'requires like every duty, if it is to be done right, the fear and love of God.[39]

By the Second World War, anxieties about nurses' body work with male patients had not abated, but exhortations to nursing as a Christian duty did not apply in the same way any more. As one nurse who trained at St Thomas' Hospital admitted, students in 1938 were told to 'polish their brasses to the glory of God'; in 1941 such edicts had lost their power.[40] The Second World War therefore witnessed concerns regarding the behaviour of women in general and a reduction in the ideology of 'nursing-as-sacrifice'. It is likely that nurses felt injunctions to silence on body care were still worth obeying in order to reduce the potential for 'pollution' created by intimate access to the male body.[41]

Nursing may have been the epitome of women's work, but that did not make its involvement with naked men easy to manage. In her exploration of 'dirty' 'body care' that contributes to the most fundamental aspects of nursing work, Jocalyn Lawler demonstrates that it is body work in particular that is 'left behind' as one becomes more senior. The work therefore is perceived as neither skilled nor desirable even by the nursing profession itself.[42] Nor is this disgust at young women's body work with men confined to nurses themselves. Penny Starns maintains that Indian and African male staff regarded with incredulity the body work that female nurses on active service overseas performed.[43] Radloff admitted causing great offence in India when she carried out intimate care on a local man, commenting that she was told that white women could not be seen doing physical work. Bodily care was the province of the male orderly.[44]

Morgan's letters to her mother may be unusually frank in their reporting of the war, the misery and desperation it caused and her work within it, but her reflections on body care are both rare and brief. In a letter in May 1941 she lists 'dressings, blanket baths, admissions, talking, cheering, teasing, ordering, the day goes by until tea'.[45] Then in another letter, in July 1943, she wrote of the need to 'wash their sweaty faces'.[46] In August 1944 she described the very 'primitive' hospital, 'and at the moment there's the almost *usual* water shortage, but we get along very well and the boys never object to going dirty that's one blessing!'[47] Sisters Geraldine Edge and Mary Johnston's account of their experiences on the hospital carrier ship HMHS *Leinster* is just as careful in its description of the body care given to young men: 'We set to work on the wounded that had just come on; so far they had only field dressings and were badly in need of attention. Four days growth of beard and a corresponding accumulation of dirt had to be removed.'[48] In her diary written aboard HMS *Dorsetshire* off the coast at Tobruk, Sister Helen Luker's description of a convoy of patients admitted to her ward is no more detailed, 'we feed, tuck them up for the night, not half of them get washed, some are very ill'.[49] Sister Jessie Wilson is equally brief in her narrative of the care given to Greek soldiers as they arrived from fighting in Albania. Moreover, she has a chaperone: 'Mac, the Australian orderly and I got them into bed, bathed and fed them.'[50] Yet this momentary description of bodily care is stark against the graphic description of one particular patient's head wound. Arguably, it is the nature of body care and not the horrors of war nursing per se that is problematic: 'We came to one old Cypriot, his head covered with blood. I started to cut away some of the hair, when I discovered a huge scalp wound and pieces of bone in his hair. A piece of shrapnel had pierced his tin hat, and the top of his skull had been smashed like an eggshell.'[51] Sister Mogg and an anonymous TANS sister who were both in the Middle Eastern desert war in 1942 provide similar succinct descriptions of bodily care. Mogg wrote: 'the minor cases who were tired and caked with sand, had their wounds dressed and were then washed, fed and rested'.[52] The anonymous TANS sister's testimony, whilst it is as brief in its allusion to bodily care, does begin to develop the understanding that the combatants needed a more supportive care regime and not just one built on efficiency:

> the patients were straight from the front line, and arrived tired, dirty, unshaven and very hungry, and some of them with very nasty wounds. They would come every day about lunch time, and we would feed and clean them as best we could … with such great numbers we were able to do very little for them apart from the bare necessities.[53]

During her posting to the Middle East, Wilson worked on a surgical ward: 'All walking wounded were sent to the bath whenever possible. How they appreciated their first hot bath for months! Stretcher cases were bed-bathed … Sometimes the men fell asleep as we were bathing them, just worn out.'[54] Many of the narratives of Second World War nurses' fundamental care practices are reminiscent of their trained nurse predecessors in the previous conflict. Personal hygiene care by nurses does not change. In *Containing Trauma*, Christine Hallett cites a British-trained nurse: 'You could not distinguish a feature, and he was caked in mud and blood.'[55] Like the TANS sister and Wilson above, the writings of trained nurses such as Kate Luard and Alice Fitzgerald articulate a non-romantic vision of the soldier-patient's

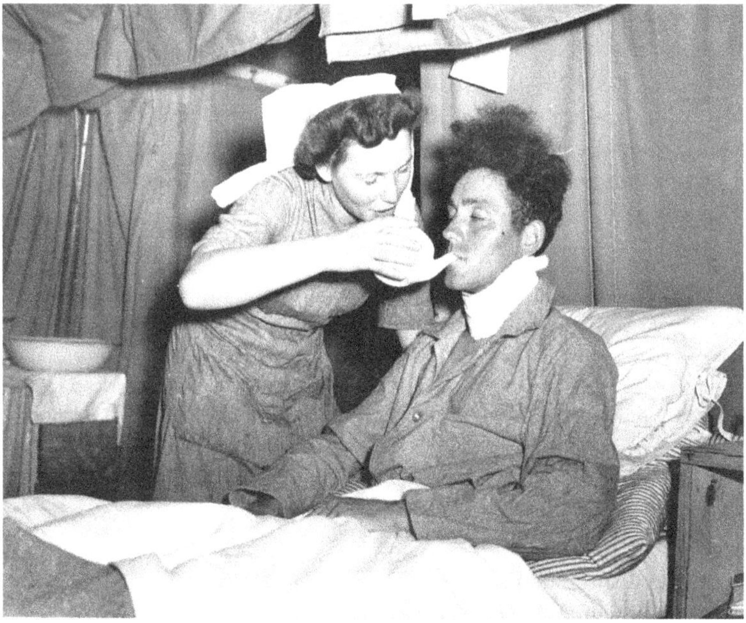

2 Italy 5th Army, assisting the helpless, 1944. Securing sufficient nutritious food for soldier-patients demanded nurses' ingenuity. Physical impairments caused by war injuries added to the burden of ensuring that men were well fed.

suffering. In her memoir, Fitzgerald wrote that she had not written her diary for propaganda purposes or publication, but to provide 'day by day account of events in a war mad world'.[56]

The best-known narratives of the First World War come from volunteer nurses, such as Vera Brittain, Mary Borden and Ellen La Motte, women who saw themselves as authors and as witnesses to war; they are far more poetic, more romantic.[57] In *The Backwash of War*, La Motte described the care of the dying soldier: 'The little stranger Rochard, with one blind, red eye that stared into Hell, the Hell he had come from. And one white, dying eye that showed his hold on life, his brief short hold. The nurse cared for him very gently, very conscientiously, very skilfully.'[58] Most of the Second World War nurses who wrote diaries, letters and other unpublished personal testimony were trained nurses before they were writers. Their narratives are therefore quite different, more realistic and prosaic. There are, however, exceptions to this. McBryde's description of the care given to a soldier too badly wounded to move provides an unusually detailed narrative of intimate nursing care. Furthermore, as it was written for publication, many years after the end of the conflict, it is evocative of the writings of the volunteer nurses of the First World War – loving and elegiac. This vignette, as with Wilson's above, is also more detailed because both men were so ill that any image of sexual tension was voided:[59]

> Gently, we eased him out of his jacket and what was left of his trousers, still caked in mud … I cradled him firmly to me while Joan soaped and gently sponged his back, all reddened and pitted with bits of earth and grass. Then she rolled up the soiled blanket from underneath him and laid a clean one alongside. In this position, we drew on one sleeve of a pyjama jacket and rolled him smoothly over the hump of blankets to Joan. Swiftly now, because he was lying on his injured leg, I pulled away the dirty blanket straightened the clean one eased on the rest of his pyjama jacket, then let him slip back gently on to a cool, clean pillow.[60]

McBryde maintained that it took 40 minutes to provide the care for this one patient. Her memoir, originally published in 1979, 34 years after the end of the war, was clearly meant to create sympathy for the patient. The use of the word 'gently' three times in the recollection demands a sense of pathos from the reader and removes the spectre of impropriety. So too does the presence of two nurses at the bedside, providing as they do a chaperone for each other. Furthermore in the 30-year hiatus between the Second World War and the publication of the memoir, attitudes to women and their relations to men had changed substantially.

Despite the paucity of detailed descriptions of intimate care,[61] the testimonies do point to such care being proffered, but often when associated with more clinical aspects of nursing work.[62] Sister Catherine Hutchinson worked on a hospital ship transporting patients back to Britain, many of whom had been fighting in Italy. She recalled one sergeant who, she said, 'greatly aroused my sympathy because he gave me the impression that he knew the seriousness of his condition'.[63] He had a bladder infection which had given rise to a high fever and was incontinent of faeces. His extensive and distressing physical problems required three to four people to support his hygiene needs, necessitating the involvement of non-nursing staff to help, including the Church of England padre. Not only is the bodily care of patients therefore passed on to others, in this case a minister, who were less likely to raise the spectre of impropriety, but also bodily care is subsumed into narratives of clinical work; work that appears to be less intimate and more professional.

The description by Radloff of treating scabies is perhaps the only time in the extensive primary sources used for the study that the 'naked' male is mentioned, and here it is not as part of washing and comfort care but as part of clinical nursing: 'As always one could only marvel at the patience of the patients with their acceptance of much ignomony [*sic*] and degradation. They had to stand completely naked while we sisters carried out this horrible procedure. I had been depersonalised – it must have been so much worse for them.'[64] What she apparently does not consider here is that the soldier has already also been dehumanised. As Emma Newlands argues, 'The very first step in the army's training regime was to establish control over the recruit's body.'[65] In a war, the purpose of which is to injure and destroy human beings,[66] the only purpose of the soldier is to 'fight even when the situation seemed hopeless'.[67] By recognising the ignominy of the treatment and the degradation the soldiers must have felt, rather than focusing on diagnosis and treatment regimes,[68] Radloff had already acknowledged the personhood of soldiers and was realising the potential for a more humanitarian nursing practice that could temper the destruction of war and recover men. If, in the narratives of body care, nurses constantly manoeuvred themselves around the desire to bear witness to men's suffering, expectations that nurses would be kindly and the ever-present fears of moral and physical pollution, other aspects of their nursing work were more simple. Feeding is mother-work; there are no ambiguities and no questions of suspect sexual knowledge by young single women. The ease with which the nurses identify this work in their testimonies is evidence of this.

Feeding work

The provision of nutritious food was the ideal of womanly care and gave nurses, as it did many women at home, a sense of worth. Julia Brock and colleagues argue that not only did the women themselves take pride in this role, but the allied governments rapidly developed an appreciation of the 'power of women' in managing wartime rations and restricting waste.[69] In the difficult years of the 1930s, food and its price had become a political motive for women. Nineteen-thirties' feminism may have reasserted traditional family structures,[70] but many women were more aware of their position and their value in the home. The political import of food was so significant that, according to Julie Gottleib, Edith Summerskill changed her general election campaign to focus on women's issues, including the price of food, rather than on foreign policy. In this move Summerskill was to be vindicated, despite fears that the expectation that women would concern themselves with the domestic rather than global politics could be used to maintain the status quo.[71] It was Summerskill's campaign grounded in the ideology of separate spheres, one that located women in the domestic space, that won her her seat.[72] Health inequalities that arose from poor nutrition may have played into the hands of those who wished for working-class girls' and women's education to focus on domestic skills, but they also identified the importance of good nutrition to create a fitter, stronger soldier.[73] Like women in general, nurses were aware of the value of good nutrition for health and healing, and their essential role in its provision.

The interwar stress on the importance of motherhood and the virtues of organising the domestic space was used by nurses on active service overseas to legitimise their position and demonstrate both their thoughtful care and their ingenuity. Whilst there was substantial research into the nutritional status of foods and what type of foods were needed to maintain and restore health,[74] few medical officers would have had either the interest in or the knowledge about preparation and administration of food to the sick. It was left to the nursing staff to ensure that food appropriate for healing was created out of monotonous field army rations.[75] Mark Harrison considers the appalling diets that caused debility and deficiency diseases,[76] and Kevin Brown identifies the severe lack of food for those imprisoned in Japanese camps.[77] However, as patient feeding was not part of the medical officers' work, neither focuses on the practical matters of ensuring adequate nutrition.

As historians of nursing have become more interested in the fundamental aspects of nursing work, they have started to contribute significantly to this crucial yet neglected study. The preparation and administration of food for the sick had been a part of nurse training since the developments of schools of nursing in the nineteenth century. Furthermore, nurses saw this work as involving skilled decision making, rather than being a simple domestic task.[78] In the absence of drug therapies, it was often the only method of supporting recovery.[79] As Charlotte Dale argues, during the Second Anglo-Boer War (1899–1902) the provision of 'food, fluids and palliatives'[80] was the only treatment regimen for typhoid.[81] Although by the Second World War, TAB (typhoid-paratyphoid A and B) vaccination against typhoid was given to all those on active service and there had been some success with using sulphaguanidine against the disease,[82] nursing staff were still required to be hypervigilant with the dietary regimes for those infected. Such care was not always easy with rations of 'bully beef and biscuits'.[83] Patient feeding had a dual role for nurses in war. It was understood as vital for their patients' physical and psychological recovery and it provided nurses with an area of autonomous practice.[84] Thus, despite advances in drug therapy, the feeding aspect of nursing work in the Second World War remained critical to nurses if they were to promote the well-being and recovery of those in their care.

Unlike the caution taken by nurses in their personal testimonies apropos body care, nutritional support and feeding work are frequent themes for discussion, including both the quantity and quality as well as where to access food and how to select and prepare appropriate food. Even after the advent of penicillin, there remained a firm belief in the absolute importance of patients receiving nutritious food in order to combat disease and injury. As late as February 1945 the Royal Air Force (RAF) was still laying stress on food to prevent illness and support recovery rather than reduce patients' 'vitality' with drugs.[85]

Access to nutritious food was, however, a recurring if not perpetual problem for nurses and their patients, especially in more mobile hospital units. One nursing sister recalled the people arriving in droves and the nurses having to forage for food to feed them during the evacuation from France in the summer of 1940.[86] Jean Bowden wrote of a Sister Leyland during the evacuation, who had a CCS with about 1,200 combatant patients and 'not much to give them except Bovril'. Allowing for artistic licence in her text, the limited access to food for the ill and injured was clearly severe.[87] According to Sister Leeming, food in a tented desert hospital was 'scant and indifferent',[88] and Sister Nell Jarrett complained that instead of nursing, she spent her time trying to organise sufficient food.[89] Despite these problems, nurses, orderlies, quartermasters and the cooks with whom they worked were usually able to provide more nutritious and plentiful food-stuffs in hospital than had been available on the battlefield.[90] When stationed on HMHS *Leinster* off the coast of Iceland, Matron R.G. Moffat was impressed by the 'great deal of trouble [that] was taken by the chief steward to arrange meals', in spite of the hospital ship's being 'frozen in'.[91] Sister E. Alty commended the quartermaster sergeant during the evacuation from France in 1940 for not only procuring food, but also cooking it himself,[92] although such praise was not universal. Sister Emily Soper maintained that she experienced difficulties in obtaining food for their patients because the quartermasters would not allow them access.[93] It is not clear whether this refusal to support the nurses' patient feeding was gendered or part of military tribalism, but even though there were evidently many exceptions, historians of wartime nursing have identified it as a problem in all wars.[94]

Once in a base hospital with improved, if still sometimes restricted, access to food and water, nurses worked hard to encourage adequate nutrition to improve their soldier-patients' health.[95] Sister Travis's experiences in the desert were of reasonable food and well cooked, but monotonous and not always suitable for those who required special diets, such as in cases of jaundice.[96] Bolton, who nursed the Chindits in India, was only too aware of the difficulties of feeding those with dysentery when their stomachs could not cope with food: 'They would ask for a generous helping, start to eat avidly, then put their plate down with regret, their stomachs not able to cope with anything stronger than milk dishes and eggs.'[97] Sister Jessie Higgins of the Princess Mary's Royal Air Force Nursing Service (PMRAFNS) in Burma in 1944 described being confronted with:

> Nothing but sickness with us, really … We had awful problems getting ill boys to eat and drink because the food was absolutely ghastly and of course you couldn't get any oranges or lemons, the only thing you could get was limes, and that [*sic*] very few and far between, we used to barter them for pilchards in tomato sauce, with the villagers. The limes were very precious and these very ill boys … we had lots of boys with minor heart conditions, a result of dysentery or typhoid. Well we used to have two great big enamel

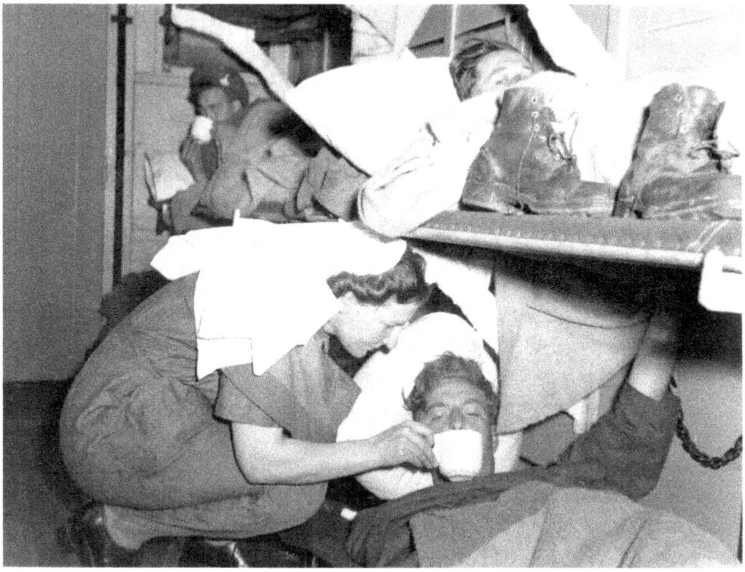

3 Wounded arriving back from Normandy on board a hospital train, 7 June 1944. Providing adequate nutrition for patients on moving hospital trains was not an easy task.

> jugs, one was blue and one was white, and we used to make squash drink (*limeade*) – in one and keep that for the really ill boys that needed the vitamin C.[98]

In response to the needs of their soldier-patients, nursing sisters realised that the physical benefits of nutritious and varied food was only one aspect of patient feeding. They also appreciated the psychological benefits of food and meal-times as methods of rehabilitating men for the return to battle or civilian life. Sister Luker wrote of the joy of 'really spoiling our patients with extra supplies of drinks, food, chocolate'.[99] Sister Mary Bond was posted to the Middle East in the winter of 1940. In her memoir she maintained that one of the most important aspects of her work in supporting the healing of her combatant patients was to 'make their meals as enjoyable as I could, sometimes I would make extras from eggs bought from local people. A favourite was scrambled eggs with cheese cooked on a "Dixie" lid on a primus stove in the ward.'[100] Morgan had one very young soldier in her care who would not eat any of the food they usually gave their sick patients, 'all the things we perjure our souls to procure for him, but mutters in a weak voice, "me [*sic*] mother makes OXO for me when I feel sick at home"'.[101]

The image of the nurse as mother feeding her 'flock' was a more palatable narrative than the hands of the nurse on the male body. Yet, as with the use of clinical nursing to identify scientific skills, some testimonies present feeding work as a clinical task as well as a homely one. This can be seen most particularly when considering those patients who had facial surgery. The data suggest not only dedicated care on the part of the nurses, but also considerable skill and improvisation:

> Great care is taken over the patient's diet. The calorie balance is carefully studied. Diet is varied as much as possible. Masks are worn during the treatment and while feeding the patients. The rubber protected spouted feeders are thoroughly cleansed and sterilised before and after use. Special attention is given to the hygiene of the mouth, strictly aseptic precautions are observed.[102]

The importance of patient feeding and the vital role that nurses played in this work was thus written into the lexicon of nursing in the Second World War. Whether appropriate medication was available or not, the acknowledgement that good nutrition was crucial to healing provided the military nurse with an area of practice that she could call her own.[103] Nursing sisters needed to use considerable skills of negotiation, improvisation and ingenuity to ensure that their patients received adequate and appropriate nutrition. These skills necessitated extensions of both their interpersonal skills and technological capabilities,[104] which were developed not only in response to feeding, but also in more clinical work, such as pain management.

Rehumanising men: healing skills in pain and death

Managing combatants' pain

The physical and mental trauma inflicted by the battles of the Second World War assaulted men's bodies.[105] Nurses' skills and humane responses to distress are seen in their ability to respond to this trauma, so that rapid detection of physical and emotional pain, or impending death, enabled appropriate and supportive care. Assistant Matron

Gillespie was posted to a hospital in Cairo just as the battle casualties from the Western Desert started arriving: 'Meanwhile, the Matron, divisional Sisters and I were giving the men tea and cigarettes. Often we picked out men who seemed especially sick or in great pain, and these we got through to the wards straight away.'[106] Whilst Gillespie demonstrates the important clinical role of nurses as part of a triage process,[107] she also showed awareness of the vital importance of the fundamental aspects of nursing care, most particularly the need for kindness, rest, nutrition and pain relief.

Santanu Das maintains that emotional and physical pain are almost impossible to discern as an outsider, as they 'stubbornly [resist] objectification in language'.[108] Yet nursing sisters were required to recognise, assess and manage their patients' pain in order to enable the healing process. Pain associated with the combatants' injuries and diseases therefore provided them with significant work. Bright's elegiac description of the damage physical pain does to recovery helps the reader to understand the importance of the provision of good pain relief:

> Pain made a patient self-absorbed, querulous, difficult, impatient, and unjust ... Pain alters the very best of characters, and should not be tolerated. At night there is a greater deal of concentration on pain, because there is little to distract the mind, and by day it forbids the simple pleasures of eating, dozing, thinking; it pursues its own course so relentlessly that it leaves a stunted, perverted mind, and a longing to die.[109]

Given the centrality of pain to the experience of many soldiers, it seems odd that not more discussion is given to this aspect of care in histories of the Second World War. It may be that this is partly because the administration of analgesia is a nursing role and thus omitted from explorations of military medicine. Although there are more discussions of the administration of pain relief in wartime nursing histories, these are still not extensive.[110] It is possible that the absence from the historical canon was in response to soldiers' fears of being considered 'weak' or malingering, or fear of being a 'bad patient'.[111] Joanna Bourke maintains there was a concern amongst soldiers that admissions of pain would bring ridicule from the ward sister and increase the work of the nurse.[112] The point of war is to kill and destroy the enemy; in order for this to happen, 'the primary move strove to reduce human agency to that of impersonal, mechanical "effectives" or "non-effectives"'.[113] In such a system pain can be seen only as the 'foe', something to be fought at all costs.[114] Certainly there were senior members of the military, such as Orde Wingate, who believed that pain could be blocked by the mind.[115] Such attitudes would have meant that some soldiers would have fought hard to deny their pain to their superiors.[116]

The transformation of the civilian male into a machine of war, coupled with an ideology that firmly maintained that the purpose of men in war was to protect women, demanded a similar stoicism when the soldier-patient came face to face with the female nurse as when he faced the military man.[117] Ana Carden-Coyne argues that to 'scream in pain, to express pain, was to act like a woman or child, and therefore invite feminization or infantilization'. Pain is bound with fear, and to express pain is to admit fear and therefore abandon the masculine self.[118] The gender dynamics in the relationships between the medical staff and patients in a military hospital in the First World War suggest a culture of manliness.[119] Twenty years later, in the Second World War, the gendered relationship between the female nurse and her combatant patient also appears to have required the soldier to retain his masculinity in order to perpetuate the belief in men's protective role.

In contrast to the limited discussions of pain in the histories of war, the frequency with which soldiers' pain is discussed in the nurses' own testimonies suggests that they placed significant importance on this aspect of nursing care. One sister wrote of the dreadful state of the Greek soldiers: 'mostly cases of frost-bite. They arrived from the hills of Albania in a terrible state, usually having travelled about seven days … drugs were administered to those in pain and the urgent cases of gangrenous limbs were operated upon. Most of the patients slept and slept and slept.'[120] Jean Bowden wrote of a train full of British and allied wounded. One RAF officer, 'was in a shocking state – severe burns', but his greatest concern was to keep his 'wings' as they cut him out of his uniform.[121] The nurses administered morphia and the pilot 'slept a little under Sister Davies' watchful eye'.[122] Another QA wrote to Dame Katharine Jones of her night on the casualty ward on Gibraltar: 'It was a never-to-be-forgotten experience, going from bed to bed re-packing wounds, applying tannic acid to burns, giving injections of morphia and laying out the dead.'[123] One of Hutchinson's patients was described as being in 'considerable pain' that was so bad he was administered the barbiturate intravenous pentothal. Although Hutchinson described his death from the cumulative effects of the drug, there is no reference to his reactions to his pain.[124] Nevertheless, in this and other explorations of caring for combatants in pain, it is clear that such work exacted considerable emotional labour on the part of the nursing sisters.

The stoicism in the face of pain meant that its accurate assessment and management was problematic. McBryde recalled the 'ultimate challenge' of caring for Australian soldiers whose denial of pain created an additional complexity to the provision of pain relief: 'some of them suffered dreadful pain but never complained'. She described how Sister Joan Wilson would let the Australians brave their pain until she felt 'that things had gone far enough'; she would then insist that they receive analgesia, but even at that point they would often refuse.[125] Much of the primary data related to pain management is in fact about German patients' pain, although there is no indication of why this should be. The care of prisoners of war (POWs) could be a significant challenge to the nursing and medical staff and not all were keen to offer German POWs the same care that they provided to their allied patients.[126] Margaret Thomas recalled a sister who would not give her German patient sufficient morphia, despite his 'bad shoulder injury and his penis was shattered, he was an awful mess and she wouldn't give him any [morphia]. If she [the sister in charge] had gone off duty, I would have given him some, but she wouldn't give him any and she was in charge.'[127] Significantly, perhaps, Thomas was in a military hospital on the home front; on active service overseas nurses seemed to take a more sympathetic attitude to POWs. Narratives that consider the care of enemy patients' pain therefore offer a different dimension to nurses' work and suggest that for some, humanitarianism was just as important as patriotism, especially when the soldiers' responses to pain were similar to those of British and Dominion soldiers.

The belief that those of northern and western European stock were more able to manage pain was, as Joanna Bourke argues, part of the pseudo-science of racial difference prevalent in the middle years of the twentieth century.[128] Thus, even when patients were the enemy, their worth as northern Europeans meant that they were considered morally superior and appreciated for their ability 'to restrain their emotions'. However, this, coupled with language difficulties, made the work of nurses challenging. Sister Evelyn Potter nursed German POWs towards the end of the war: 'I remember one German particularly and he was an ex-SS guard. He used to sit bolt upright in bed and he used to have bouts of severe pain and we only knew when his bed shook.'[129] Elizabeth Kyle's description of a nurse caring for a German general illustrates the nursing skills required to diagnose pain and provide relief without raising concerns of limited bravery. According to Kyle, the nursing sister 'knew better than to offer sympathy or ask irritating questions', as the general was clearly in pain, but would not admit to it. Instead she allowed the conversation to develop on common ground, discussing the nature of obligation by soldiers and their duties in war, whilst administering the required morphine.[130]

Not all soldiers', German or allied, responses to pain were stoic, nor was all pain physical. However, the identification of those who could and would cry out in pain is usually in descriptions of the very young, thus softening the need for manly behaviour. On 5 July 1944 a convoy of Canadian casualties arrived at Morris's hospital in Normandy: 'There were charred bodies everywhere', and although she acknowledged that some did indeed lie quietly dying, others were 'screaming with pain'. She continued, 'We gave them morphia and more morphia and watched helplessly as they died … they were all so young and frightened.'[131] Radloff recalled:

> Some died on stretchers … but a few could be rendered fit for active service. This was almost the worst part – that a young man who had been helped to recover was so terrified that he cried and begged to be spared a return to the slaughter and carnage. But back he went – and again I do not know what happened to him.[132]

The administration of morphia was a nursing duty in civilian hospitals in Britain. However, on active service overseas the need to both administer and prescribe became part of nurses' armoury of skills, with nurses making rapid decisions on the need for pain relief without recourse to medical support.[133] One TANS sister in the Middle East described the arrival of nearly 100 German POWs: 'I had to use morphia at my own discretion, there was nobody about to order and check all the time and many of them were in agony.'[134]

Having not been trained to prescribe and knowing that it was outside the remit of nursing work, this would have taken considerable risk and courage on her part. Furthermore, the uses of morphia in war zones were wider than in a civilian hospital. Luker recalled administering analgesia for pain and to support dangerously ill patients more generally. On 24 December she described how one patient 'nearly dies at 1am, but coramine, then later, morphia restore him somewhat, but his pulse is 160–176'.[135]

Death and dying

The exigencies of war meant that not all patients could be saved, and thus morphia was used not only to restore health but also to support a patient's dignified death. The development of more human-centred practices meant that nurses established a closeness to their combatant patients and then had to watch them die in what was considered 'the ultimate sacrifice'.[136] This personalisation of death was sometimes achieved at both personal and professional cost for nurses, realising as they did their impotence in its presence: 'surely three o'clock in the morning approaches the very bottom of time? To mourn seems the natural thing to do; a dying man dies … while the professional calm and dignity of a nurse become as nothing.'[137] Sister Iris Hooper was posted to a forward CCS in the latter months of the war. Writing for the *Medical Gazette* in June 1945 she stated: 'By far the greatest emotional strain was caused by being audience to the domestic and personal side of a life fast ebbing from one who seemed to have so much to live for, so much to hope for, so many ambitions to fulfil, but yet, wounded beyond repair, unable now to carry on the fight to live.'[138]

Sister Francie Brown wrote to her sisters in August 1944 of a patient she had 'specialed'.[139] His health had been improving and he was to be evacuated, then the night before his arranged departure, 'he woke at midnight – called me, + just died in three minutes. Oh I was upset – it was terrible + so unexpected. Since then I have heard from his wife + mother … It makes me feel I'll never write to relatives again.'[140] Hutchinson recalled one patient who was escorted home to Wales so that he could see his wife and home before he died. On arrival he was so ill that he was sent directly to the nearest military hospital:

> When they got there Sister S. watched helplessly as numerous American doctors descended on him and made rapid decisions to operate on him at once. A message had been sent to his wife when the ship docked, and she was on her way to see him. So Sister S. begged them to delay until she arrived. They told her the operation was too urgent … she heard he had died almost as soon as he was anaesthetised. We were all stunned.[141]

The sadness with which the full story of her Welsh patient is told contrasts with the final brief sentence. The process of caring for the very ill is a legitimate nursing narrative, but once death occurs nurses need to move on in order to manage their emotions. Despite the clear emotional trials of caring for the dying, nursing sisters would have been obligated to grieve silently and unobtrusively in a system that 'privileged stoicism in the face of loss'.[142] In a war zone where death was a common occurrence, to be incapacitated by it would have hindered nurses' abilities to care for the living.

Conclusion

The nurses who went to war between 1939 and 1945 took with them a lexicon of nursing skills and practices that enabled them to manage combatants' physical care. Yet many soon realised this was not sufficient to heal their soldier-patients; a more individual mode of nursing was needed that located their patient as a person, not an object for treatment. Body work, feeding, pain relief and support for the dying were central to the work of the nurse. They were also deeply gendered practices that required skilled negotiation on active service overseas, exacerbated by the closer relationships that were developed between nurse and patient. Body and hygiene work were the backbone of the nurse's day. Away from the close supervision of the civilian hospital system, they raised difficult questions in relation to the handling of male bodies by single young women. Nutrition and feeding were quintessentially linked to womanhood and the mother-role. However, the expertise required on active service demanded that nurses should have significant authority not only over their soldier-patients' feeding but also over access to the food-stuffs they deemed appropriate. The care of physical and emotional pain was rendered highly complex in a world where men should not admit to frailty – the masculine space of war. Military nurses therefore needed to develop both tact and clinical awareness in order to determine pain and manage it, frequently without medical support. In the absence of medical colleagues, the development of clinical skills shifted these highly feminine nursing practices to a more masculine mode. This new manner of nursing meant that the nursing sisters increasingly worked autonomously and within the realms of scientific medicine. Furthermore, without senior support, the QAs needed to cultivate their skills of ingenuity and improvisation so as to manage the multiple challenges of active service.

Notes

1 Anonymous, 'War – what it means to the nurse', *Nursing Mirror and Midwives' Journal* (2 September 1939): 755.

2 This book is about the war work and experiences of the Army nursing service in the Second World War. Although the TANS had been its own nursing service since its inception in 1908, it was merged with the QAs for the duration of the war. Thus for the purposes of the work, the QAs, their Reservists and the TANS will all come under the auspices of the QAs, military or Army nursing service, as they did for the war. Nicola Tyrer, *Sisters in Arms: British Army Nurses Tell their Story* (London: Phoenix, 2008), 17. See Anne Summers for an analysis of the Haldane Reforms and the foundation of the Territorial Army and TANS. Anne Summers, *Angels and Citizens: British Women as Military Nurses, 1854–1914* (Newbury: Threshold Press, 2000), 206–8. Although Dame Katharine Jones was Matron-in-Chief of the QAs, it is clear that she considered the TANS as much a part of her responsibility as she did the QAs. In an article in *Nursing Times* on 27 January 1945, she stated, 'I have done my best to militarize the QAIMNS and the TANS'. Dame Katharine Jones, 'QAIMNS professional and military status', *Nursing Times* (27 January 1945): 60. For a full discussion of Dame Katharine Jones' militarising mission, see Penny Starns, 'Fighting militarism? British nursing during the Second World War', in Roger Cooter, Mark Harrison and Steve Sturdy (eds), *War, Medicine and Modernity* (Stroud: Sutton Publishing, 1998).

3 QAIMNS, 'War diary: Volume I' (1 to 30 September 1939), 1.9.39, The National Archives (hereafter TNA), WO 177/14.

4 For a useful and helpful discussion on the early difficulties regarding nurses' access to male bodies, see Mary Poovey, *Uneven Developments: The Ideological Work of Gender in Mid-Victorian England* (Chicago: University of Chicago Press, 1988) and Alison Bashford, *Purity and Pollution: Gender, Embodiment and Victorian Medicine* (Basingstoke: Macmillan Press, 1998).

5 For a discussion on the difficulties in creating an artistry of nursing see Jane Brooks and Christine E. Hallett, 'Introduction: The practice of nursing and the exigencies of war', in Jane Brooks and Christine E. Hallett (eds), *One Hundred Years of Nursing Wartime Practices, 1854–1953* (Manchester: Manchester University Press, 2015), 6.

6 Cynthia Toman, *An Officer and a Lady: Canadian Military Nursing and the Second World War* (Vancouver: University of British Columbia Press, 2007), 52.

7 Male nurses were not entitled to relative rank or commissioned officer status after 1941 as their female colleagues were. Those that existed were employed in the other ranks.

8 F.A.E. Crew, 'The Army medical services', in Arthur Salusbury MacNalty and W. Frankin Mellor (eds), *Medical Services in War: The Principal Medical Lessons of the Second World War* (London: HMSO, 1968), 81.

9 Ann Radloff, "Going to Gooseberry Beach: Travels and adventures of a nursing Sister', 1, Imperial War Museum Private Papers (hereafter IWM) Documents.147

10 Brenda McBryde, *A Nurse's War* (Saffron Walden: Cakebread Publications, 1993), 86.

11 Agnes Kathleen Dunbar Morgan, 'My dearest mother', letter 57 (August 1943), Central Mediterranean Force (hereafter CMF), 4, in 'Still with the lamp: letters to my mother by an army nursing sister'. Egypt – North Africa – Sicily – Italy, 1941–1944, IWM Documents 16686.

12 Michael Ondaatje,*The English Patient* (London: Bloomsbury, 1992), 15.

13 Morgan, 'My dearest mother', letter 23: written and sent at a much later date for reasons of security, Middle East Force (hereafter MEF), 1.

14 Julie Fairman and Patricia D'Antonio have recently challenged nurses to see 'the patient beneath the machines', suggesting that this personal and humane aspect of nursing work retains its difficulties. Julie Fairman and Patricia D'Antonio, 'Reimagining nursing's place in the history of clinical practice', *Journal of the History of Medicine and Allied Health Sciences* 63, 4 (2008): 438.

15 Radloff, 'Going to Gooseberry Beach', 9.

16 Angela Bolton, *The Maturing Sun: An Army Nurse in India 1942–45* (London: Headline, 1986), 79.

17 Sheri Tesseyman, 'Complex alliance: A study of relationships between nursing and medicine in Britain and the United States of America, 1860–1914' [unpublished PhD] (Manchester: University of Manchester, 2013), 259; Kathryn McPherson, *Bedside Matters: The Transformation of Canadian Nursing, 1900–1990* (Toronto: Oxford University Press Canada, 1996), 54.

18 It should be noted that not all soldiers were heterosexual. Tommy Dickinson argues that the war was a liberating time for many homosexual men. It was, he maintains, a time when being camp could be both tolerated and enjoyed,

if it remained 'furtive'. Tommy Dickinson, *'Curing Queers': Mental Nurses and their Patients, 1935–74* (Manchester: Manchester University Press, 2015), 42.

19 Toman, *An Officer and a Lady*, 4.

20 Harrison, Mark, *Medicine and Victory: British Military Medicine in the Second World War* (Oxford: Oxford University Press, 2004), 212.

21 Joanna Bourke, *Dismembering the Male: Men's Bodies, Britain and the Great War* (London: Reaktion Books, 1996), 38.

22 Ana Carden-Coyne argues that in the hospital wards in the First World War, the spectre of sexual frisson was ever present. Whilst attitudes had changed in the intervening years, anxieties had not completely abated. See Chapter 4, 'Provocative wounds: Sociality and intimacy in war hospitals', in Ana Carden-Coyne, *The Politics of Wounds: Military Patients and Medical Power in the First World War* (Oxford: Oxford University Press, 2014).

23 Phil Goodman, '"Patriotic femininity": Women's morals and men's morale during the Second World War', *Gender and History* 10, 2 (1998): 278–93.

24 Sonya O. Rose, *Which People's War? National Identity and Citizenship in Britain, 1939–1945* (Oxford: Oxford University Press, 2003, Kindle edition), loc. 2118.

25 Gerard J. DeGroot, '"Lipstick on her nipples, cordite in her hair": Sex and romance among British servicewomen during the Second World War', in Gerard J. DeGroot and Corinna Peniston-Bird, *A Soldier and a Woman* (Abingdon: Taylor and Francis, 2014), 110.

26 Martha L. Hall, Belinda T. Orzada and Dilia Lopez-Gydosh, 'American women's wartime dress: Sociocultural ambiguities regarding women's roles during World War II', *The Journal of American Culture* 38, 3 (2015): 237. There is a great deal written about women's wearing of trousers in the Second World War and the fears that it raised about 'gender-bending', in Britain and allied countries. See for example, Gail Braybon and Penny Summerfield, *Out of the Cage: Women's Experiences in Two World Wars* (London: Pandora, 1987); Deborah Montgomerie, 'Assessing Rosie: World War II, New Zealand women and the iconography of femininity', *Gender and History*, 8, 1 (1996): 108–32; Goodman, 'Patriotic femininity'; Jeremy A. Crang, '"Come into the Army Maud": Women, military conscription, and the Markham Inquiry', *Defence Studies* 8, 3 (2008): 381–95.

27 Corinna Peniston-Bird, 'Classifying the body in the Second World War: British men in and out of uniform', *Body and Society* 9, 4 (2003): 44.

28 Cynthia Enloe, *Does Khaki Become You? The Militarization of Women's Lives* (London: Pandora, 1988) 106–7.

29 Mary Sarnecky quotes one American officer who stated that 'the nurses know how to please them [the soldiers], how to turn them, how to fix their clothes, and then, too, I think that when a man is very sick he kind of looks to a female for comfort'. The ambiguities of the nurse 'pleasing' and

being a 'female for comfort' are not explored, but it is clear that the nurse's proximity to male combatants was one of motherliness, but imbued with questions of the sort of care she could and would provide; see Lieutenant Colonel Robert Smith, cited in Mary Sarnecky, *A History of the US Army Nurse Corps* (Philadelphia, PA: University of Pennsylvania Press, 1999), 223. In order to circumvent concerns in the civilian population, popular literature, such as the Cherry Ames books, created the image of a desexualised 'pin-up' nurse, whose purity was assured by her white uniform. Adrianne Finlay, 'Cherry Ames, disembodied nurse: War, sexuality, and sacrifice in the novels of Helen Wells', *The Journal of Popular Culture* 43, 6 (2010): 1189–206.

30 Mary Morris, 'The diary of a wartime nurse' (28 September 1944), 137, IWM Documents 4850; Mary Morris, *A Very Private Diary: A Nurse in Wartime*, ed. Carol Acton (London: Weidenfeld and Nicolson, 2014), 121.

31 Morris, 'The diary of a wartime nurse' (16 October 1944), 157; Morris, *A Very Private Diary*, 136.

32 Pam Bright, *Life in our Hands: Nursing Sister's War Experiences* (London: Pan Books, 1955), 80.

33 Kathleen Canning, 'The body as method? Reflections on the place of the body in gender history', *Gender and History* 11, 3 (1999): 500.

34 Bashford, *Purity and Pollution*, 36.

35 Anne Marie Rafferty, *The Politics of Nursing Knowledge* (London: Routledge, 1996), 19.

36 Leonore Davidoff, *Worlds Between: Historical Perspectives on Gender and Class* (Cambridge: Polity Press, 1995), 77.

37 Bashford, *Purity and Pollution*, 54.

38 Rafferty, *The Politics of Nursing Knowledge*, 28.

39 Florence Nightingale, 'Subsidiary note as to the introduction of female nursing into military hospitals in peace and in war' (Thoughts submitted as to an eventual Nurses' Provident Fund), Presented to the Secretary of State for War (London: Harrison and Son, 1858): 7.

40 Anonymous military nurse, 'Frontline Females', BBC Radio 4 (11 April 1998), British Library Sound Archive H9872/2. This two-part radio programme, introduced by Claire Rayner, involved a number of Second World War nurses. It is not possible to identify individual women in the broadcast. For a full list of participants, see bibliography. This programme played a significant role in developing primary source material for Penny Starns, *Nurses at War: Women on the Frontline, 1939–45* (Stroud: Sutton Publishing, 2000).

41 Bashford, *Purity and Pollution*.

42 Jocalyn Lawler explores this in detail in *Behind the Screens: Nursing, Somology and the Problem of the Body* (Melbourne: Churchill Livingstone, 1991), 31.

43 Starns, *Nurses at War*, 55.
44 Radloff, 'Going to Gooseberry Beach', 23–4.
45 Morgan, 'My dearest mums', letter 16 (October 1941), MEF, 2–3.
46 Morgan, 'My dearest mums', letter 55 (July 1943), MEF, 2.
47 Morgan, 'My dearest mums', letter 85 (August 1944), CMF, 1.
48 Geraldine Edge and Mary E. Johnston, *Ships of Youth: The Experiences of Two Army Nursing Sisters on Board the Hospital Carrier Leinster* (London: Hodder and Stoughton, 1945), 60.
49 Esther Helen Audrey Luker, 'Diaries from 1940–45' (Monday 14 April), IWM Documents 1274. Luker's six diaries were catalogued at the Imperial War Museum in 1985. In the preface to the private papers that accompanied them is this information: 'these notes were found among the papers of Helen Luker A.R.R.C. some years after her death in 1957'.
50 Jessie Sarah Catherine Wilson, 'We also served, 1940 …', 18, UKCHN Archive, University of Manchester. I am indebted to Jessie Wilson's family for providing me with access to this war diary and for the following biographical information. Jessie was, according to her nephew, for some unknown reason also called Joan Katherine Wilson. She spent much of her childhood in care following the death of her mother in 1914, when Jessie was only 12. Despite her impoverished childhood, Jessie trained as a nurse at the Hull Royal Infirmary and joined the TANS shortly after the outbreak of the Second World War. She died aged 46 years, on 29 July 1949, of pneumonia brought on by kidney failure and anaemia.
51 Wilson, 'We also served, 1940 …', 18.
52 L.R. Mogg, 'My work and experiences in the Middle-East. No. 64 General Hospital, Alexandria', MMM QARANC uncatalogued archive.
53 Sister TANS, 'My adventures in a CCS in the Middle East', MMM QARANC/PE/1/320/World War II.
54 Wilson, 'We who also served, 1940 …', 47.
55 Anonymous, *A War Nurse's Diary: Sketches from a Belgian Field Hospital* (New York: Macmillan, 1918), 90. Cited in Christine E. Hallett, *Containing Trauma: Nursing Work in the First World War* (Manchester: Manchester University Press, 2009), 43.
56 Alice Fitzgerald, 'Memoirs', 22. Cited in Christine E. Hallett, *Nurse Writers of the Great War* (Manchester: Manchester University Press, 2016), 112.
57 Christine E. Hallett, *Nurse Writers of the Great War* (Manchester: Manchester University Press, 2016), 8. This book contains detailed accounts of the First World War nurses who wrote of their experiences.
58 Ellen Newbold La Motte, *The Backwash of War: The Human Wreckage of the Battlefield as Witnessed by an American Hospital Nurse* (New York: G.P. Putnam's Sons, 2016), 57.
59 Testimonies from nurses do suggest pathos associated with an unmanning through injury and disability. In the recently published war diary of

Sister Joyce Ffoulkes Parry, an Australian nurse who, having been born in Wales, joined the QAs in 1940: 'Graves, a New Zealander, died there last night. In the PM today they found a lung abscess and TB lesions and amoebic dysentery. The struggle was too much for him, which we could see at first, as he was a pathetic figure'; see Rhiannon Evans (ed.), Joyce Ffoulkes Parry, *Joyce's War: The Second World War Journal of a Queen Alexandra's Imperial Military Nursing Service Nurse* (28 November 1940) (Stroud: The History Press, 2015, Kindle edition), loc. 915.

60 McBryde, *A Nurse's War*, 95

61 In neither Anna Rogers nor Jan Bassett's books on the New Zealand and Australian Army Nursing Services does nursing work feature heavily. Although they both provide some discussions of clinical and comfort nursing care, the focus is mainly on bravery and adversity; see Jan Bassett, *Guns and Brooches: Australian Army Nursing from the Boer War to the Gulf War* (Oxford: Oxford University Press, 1992) and Anna Rogers, *While You're Away: New Zealand Nurses at War, 1899–1948* (Auckland: Auckland University Press 2003).

62 Nurses have, according to Brooks and Hallett, found it easier to articulate their practice as science rather than artistry. For a wider discussion of this see Brooks and Hallett, 'Introduction: The practice of nursing and the exigencies of war', 5–6.

63 Catherine Arnold Hutchinson, 'My war and welcome to it' (March 2001), 37, IWM Documents 11950.

64 Radloff, 'Going to Gooseberry Beach', 17.

65 Emma Newlands, *Civilians into Soldiers: War, the Body and British Army Recruits, 1939–45* (Manchester: Manchester University Press, 2014), 54.

66 Joanna Bourke, *The Second World War: A People's History* (Oxford: Oxford University Press, 2001).

67 Jonathan Fennell, 'Courage and cowardice in the North African Campaign: The Eighth Army and defeat in the summer of 1942', *War in History* 20, 1 (2013): 106.

68 Karen Buhler-Wilkerson's seminal text, *No Place Like Home: A History of Nursing and Home Care in the United States* (Baltimore, MD: Johns Hopkins University Press, 2001) offers an exposition of how community visiting nurses, working alone and with patients with complex, long-term conditions, developed a relatively autonomous practice in which they increasingly realised that it was the patient and their carers' needs that should be at the forefront of the care that should be given, not the medical diagnosis. The situation for community nurses in Britain was no different, and in the inter-war years the Depression led to an increased number of patients from wide social strata and with the complexity of problems associated with poverty, overcrowding, ill-health and multiple births. For district nurses in rural areas this could be exacerbated by what was called

double or triple duty nurses; those who were nurses and midwives and, in some cases, health visitors as well. Because of this expertise, the government sought to limit district nurses from volunteering for military service. Helen M. Sweet and Rona Dougall, *Community Nursing and Primary Healthcare in Twentieth-Century Britain* (New York: Routledge, 2008), 64.

69 Julia Brock, Jennifer W. Dickey, Richard J.W. Harker and Catherine M. Lewis (eds), *Beyond Rosie: A Documentary History of Women and World War II* (Fayetteville, AK: University of Arkansas Press, 2015, Kindle edition), loc. 592. See also Gail Braybon and Penny Summerfield, *Out of the Cage: Women's Experiences in Two World Wars* (London: Pandora, 1987), 247.

70 Caine, *English Feminism*, 174.

71 Pat Thane, 'What difference did the vote make? Women in public and private life in Britain since 1918', *Historical Research* 76, 192 (2003): 277.

72 Julie V. Gottlieb, 'Munich By-elections, 1938–1939', in Julie V. Gottlieb and Richard Toye, *The Aftermath of Suffrage: Women, Gender, and Politics in Britain 1918–1945* (Basingstoke: Palgrave Macmillan, 2013), 163.

73 Newlands, *Civilians into Soldiers*, 38. There is a wealth of literature on the gendered education for domesticity in the early twentieth century, following the realisation of the poor fitness of the working man in the Second Anglo-Boer War. See most especially, Anna Davin, 'Imperialism and motherhood', *History Workshop Journal* 5 (1978): 9–65; Dorothy Porter, Part 3: 'The obligations of health in the twentieth century', in Dorothy Porter, *Health, Civilization and the State: A History of Public Health from Ancient to Modern Times* (London: Routledge, 1999); Jane Brooks, Chapter 3, 'Nursing the nation', in Jane Brooks, '"Visiting rights only": The early experience of nurses in higher education, 1918–1960' [unpublished PhD thesis] (London: London School of Hygiene and Tropical Medicine, 2005).

74 Arthur Salusbury MacNalty, 'Medical research', in Arthur Salusbury MacNalty and W. Franklin Mellor (eds), *Medical Services in War: The Principal Medical Lessons of the Second World War* (London: HMSO, 1968), 383–4.

75 Nicola Tyrer, *Sisters in Arms: British Army Nurses Tell their Story* (London: Phoenix, 2008), 155.

76 Harrison, *Medicine and Victory*, see particularly 54, 70.

77 Kevin Brown, *Fighting Fit: Health, Medicine and War in the Twentieth Century* (Stroud: The History Press, 2008, Kindle edition), loc. 5138.

78 Carol Helmstadter, 'Class, gender and professional expertise: British military nursing in the Crimean War', in Jane Brooks and Christine E. Hallett (eds), *One Hundred Years of Wartime Nursing Practices, 1854–1953* (Manchester: Manchester University Press, 2015). According to Jane Schultz, when white women took over the kitchens during the America Civil War, the importance and value of cooking 'gained prestige' through

their participation. Jane E. Schultz, *Women at the Front: Hospital Workers in Civil War America* (Chapel Hill, NC: University of North Carolina Press, 2004), 35.

79 Kirsty Harris, '"Health, healing and harmony": Invalid cookery and feeding by Australian Nurses in the Middle East in the First World War', in Jane Brooks and Christine E. Hallett (eds), *One Hundred Years of Wartime Nursing Practices, 1854–1953* (Manchester: Manchester University Press, 2015), 109.

80 Therese Connell Meehan, 'Careful nursing: A model for contemporary nursing practice', *Journal of Advanced Nursing* 44, 1 (2003): 100.

81 Charlotte Dale, 'Traversing the veldt with "Tommy Atkins": The clinical challenges of nursing typhoid patients during the Second Anglo-Boer War (1899–1902)', in Jane Brooks and Christine E. Hallett (eds), *One Hundred Years of Wartime Nursing Practices, 1854–1953* (Manchester: Manchester University Press, 2015). For further discussion of the nursing care required for those suffering from typhoid, see also Anne Summers, *Angels and Citizens: British Women as Military Nurses, 1854–1914* (Newbury: Threshold Press, 2000), 174–8.

82 E.H.R. Harries, Robert Swyer and Noel Thompson, 'Sulphanilamide in typhoid fever', *The Lancet* (10 June 1939): 1321–24; John F. Stokes, 'The present status of the sulphonamide drugs', *Nursing Times* (21 February 1942): 124–5. Penicillin was not effective against typhoid. Anonymous, 'Penicillin: Indications for its use and methods of administration', *The British Journal of Nursing* (April 1945): 39. It was not until the manufacture of chloramphenicol at the end of the 1940s that it was possible to cure both typhoid and typhus. Robert Bud, *Penicillin: Triumph and Tragedy* (Oxford: Oxford University Press, 2007), 108.

83 QAIMNS Reserve, 'The Departure of the British military hospital, Marseilles', in Ada Harrison (ed.), *Grey and Scarlet: Letters From the War Areas by Army Sisters on Active Service* (London: Hodder and Stoughton, 1944), 27.

84 Jane Brooks, 'Wartime nursing: Feeding as forgotten practice', in Sandra B. Lewenson, Annemarie McAllister and Kylie Smith (eds), *Nursing History for Contemporary Role Development* (New York: Springer, 2017); Jane Brooks, '"Uninterested in anything except food": Nurse feeding work with the liberated inmates of Bergen-Belsen', *Journal of Clinical Nursing* 21 (2012): 2963; Jane Brooks, '"The nurse stoops down for me": Nursing the liberated persons at Bergen-Belsen', in Jane Brooks and Christine Hallett (eds), *One Hundred Years of Nursing Wartime Practices, 1854–1953* (Manchester: Manchester University Press, 2015), 224.

85 J. Elsie Gordon, 'With the Nursing Sisters on the Western Front – 2. At RAF General Hospital in Brussels', *Nursing Mirror* (3 February 1945): 243, 250.

86 A Theatre Sister, 'A casualty clearing station in France, April 12th to May

29th, 1940', in Ada Harrison (ed.), *Grey and Scarlet: Letters From the War Areas by Army Sisters on Active Service* (London: Hodder and Stoughton, 1944), 52.

87 Jean Bowden, *Grey Touched with Scarlet: The War Experiences of Army Nursing Sisters* (London: Robert Hale, 1959), 402.

88 E.M. Leeming, 'My war years, 1939–1945', Wellcome Trust Collection, PP/Lee/1, 3.

89 Nell Jarrett, Diary of her desert experiences' (21 June 1942–13 January 1943) (17 October 1942), UKCHN Archive, University of Manchester.

90 There are many places in the personal testimonies where quartermasters, orderlies and cooks are praised by the nursing sisters. See for example, Catherine M. Butland, 'Army sisters in battledress or the chosen few or follow fate', 49, MMM, QARANC/PE/1/74/BUTL Box 8; E. Alty, 'Three Army sisters leave France', 5, MMM, QARANC/PE/1/321/France BEF, Box 68.

91 R.G. Moffat, 'Experiences on HMHS Leinster, November 1940-May 1941', 2, MMM, Envelope, three letters and reports, Box 68.

92 Alty, 'Three Army sisters leave France', 3.

93 Emily Soper, oral history interview by Jane Brooks on 6 September 2013.

94 See, for example, Helmstadter, 'Class, gender and professional expertise: British military nursing in the Crimean War'; 33; Harris, 'Health, healing and harmony', 111; Dale, 'Traversing the veldt with "Tommy Atkins"', 68.

95 Wilson, 'We also served', 29.

96 Mary Travis (TANS), 'General hospital in the desert: Middle East Forces', MMM QARANC, uncatalogued archive.

97 Bolton, *The Maturing Sun*, 147.

98 Jessie Higgins, oral history interview by Mary Mackie, 24 March 1999 at her home in Girton, Cambridge. Italics in the original. Jessie Higgins joined the PMRAFNS in 1939 and served with them until her retirement in 1968. For an extensive discussion of Jessie Higgins' life and work see Mary Mackie, *Sky Wards: A History of the Princess Mary's Royal Air Force Nursing Service* (London: Robert Hale, 2001).

99 Luker, 'Diaries from 1940–45', 15.

100 Mary Bond, *Wartime Experiences from the Midnight Sun to Belsen* (Cardigan: E.L. Jones and Son, 1994), 30.

101 Morgan, 'My dearest mother', letter 65 (October 1943), CMF, 1.

102 Anonymous, 'The adventures of a nursing officer (QAIMNSR) 1939–1945 and some highlights on nursing of some tropical diseases, also battle wounds. No. 9 GH, MEF', 14, MMM QARANC uncatalogued archive, MEF memoirs.

103 Penny Salter, 'Long ago and far away: A distant memory: A diary, c. 1938–1970', 124, personal archive and IWM Documents 17694.

104 Jillian MacGuire, 'Tailoring research for therapeutic nursing practice',

in Richard McMahon and Alan Pearson, *Nursing as Therapy* (2nd edn) (Cheltenham: Stanley Thorne, 1998), 157.

105 Newlands, *Civilians into Soldiers*, 17.

106 H.S. Gillespie, 'Some experiences in hospitals in the Middle East, 1939–1942', 2, MMM QARANC uncatalogued archive.

107 Triage is the process of sorting patients. At its most brutal, the process sorts patients into those who need immediate treatment to survive, those who will survive if treatment is delayed and those who will not survive despite treatment. More commonly it is the process of sorting patients who need treatment most urgently down to those who can wait. Traditionally this was a medical task, but on active service overseas it was frequently undertaken by nursing sisters.

108 Santanu Das, *Touch and Intimacy in First World War Literature* (Cambridge: Cambridge University Press, 2005), 188–9.

109 Bright, *Life in our Hands*, 62.

110 Cynthia Toman does not provide a discussion of the nursing work of pain relief, although she acknowledges the importance placed on precise drug dosages by nursing leaders. Toman, *An Officer and A Lady*, 120; Jan Bassett's discussion is one that includes concern for pain alongside the concern of Australian nurses' required evacuation from their hospital before the battle for Tobruk; see, Bassett, *Guns and Brooches*, 120.

111 Joanna Bourke, *The Story of Pain: From Prayer to Painkillers* (Oxford: Oxford University Press, 2014), 133.

112 Bourke, *The Story of Pain*, 139.

113 Joanna Bourke, 'Disciplining the emotions: Fear, psychiatry and the Second World War', in Roger Cooter, Mark Harrison and Steve Sturdy (eds), *War, Medicine and Modernity* (Stroud: Sutton Publishing, 1998), 225.

114 Bourke, *The Story of Pain*, 21.

115 Harrison, *Medicine and Victory*, 212. Orde Wingate led the 'Chindits', a multi-national allied force that engaged in a type of guerrilla warfare behind Japanese lines. He has been summarily been described as both genius and fanatic. His methods did lead to the loss of over 1,000 men. However, as Harrison suggests, Wingate's admiration of the work of Matron McGreary and his determination to evacuate men whenever possible to her hospital in Sylhet demonstrate an interest in the well-being of his troops that is not always fully appreciated; see Harrison, *Medicine and Victory*, 204.

116 According to Anne Alwis, the admission of pain is 'a state at odds with cultural conceptions of masculinity, both modern and most particularly, ancient'; see Anne P. Alwis, 'Men in pain: Masculinity, medicine and the *Miracles* of St. Artemios', *Byzantine and Modern Greek Studies* 36, 1 (2012): 2. In the mid-nineteenth century the forbearance of pain was instilled through sport and the cadet system at the public schools of Britain; see, for example, Michael Roper, 'Between manliness and masculinity: The "war"

generation" and the psychology of fear in Britain, 1914–1950', *Journal of British Studies* 44 (2005): 343–62.

117 Newlands, *Civilians into Soldiers*.

118 Carden-Coyne, *The Politics of Wounds*, 335.

119 Carden-Coyne, *The Politics of Wounds*, 336.

120 A Sister TANS, 'Greece and the Middle East', in Ada Harrison (ed.), *Grey and Scarlet: Letters From the War Areas by Army Sisters on Active Service* (London: Hodder and Stoughton, 1944), 144.

121 Bowden, *Grey Touched with Scarlet*, 23.

122 Bowden, *Grey Touched with Scarlet*, 24.

123 Sister QAIMNS Reserve, 'Gibraltar: January 1940–January1942', in Ada Harrison (ed.), *Grey and Scarlet: Letters From the War Areas by Army Sisters on Active Service* (London: Hodder and Stoughton, 1944), 136.

124 Hutchinson, 'My war and welcome to it', 34.

125 Brenda McBryde, *Quiet Heroines: Nurses of the Second World War* (London: Chatto and Windus, 1985), 129.

126 The rights of POWs, including the right to medical treatment, were (and continue to be) safeguarded by the Geneva Convention of 1929. Crew, 'The Army Medical Services', 156. However, as Harrison argues, this obligation was not always followed by the Germans, who were, unlike the Japanese, signed up to the Convention. Harrison, *Medicine and Victory*, 53. It is not known how widespread poor treatment of POWs in British hands was, although there are incidences reported which demonstrate that parity with their own men was not always shown. For example, Hutchinson's memoir recalls a debacle she had with a medical officer over the care she wanted to give to her Italian POW patients, who he felt were 'only POWs after all'. Hutchinson, 'My war and welcome to it', 62–3.

127 Margaret Thomas, oral history interview via telephone by Jane Brooks, 17 February 2014. This part of the oral history interview was clearly a disturbing one. Thomas took time over the telling of this narrative, the tragedy being compounded by her inability to do anything because of the Sister's authority. Thomas said, 'Very difficult that … It plays on my mind, it was really one of the worst things that happened.' This oral history highlights the potential dangers of the method and the absolute requirement for the interviewer to be cognisant of the potential for distress. For a detailed discussion of the dangers of oral history, see Wendy Rickard, 'Oral history – "More dangerous than therapy"? Interviewees' reflections on recording traumatic or taboo issues', *Oral History* 26, 2, 'Memory, Trauma and Ethics' (1998): 34–48.

128 Bourke, *The Story of Pain*, p. 198.

129 Evelyn Potter (pseudonym), oral history interview via telephone by Jane Brooks, 16 September 2013.

130 Elisabeth Kyle, 'Hospital in the desert', MMM QARANC Box 18.

131 Morris, 'The diary of a wartime nurse' (5 July 1944), 121; Morris, *A Very Private Diary*, 103.
132 Radloff, 'Going to Gooseberry Beach', 12.
133 A Sister, Q.AIMNS, 'An ambulance train in the evacuation from France', in Ada Harrison (ed.), *Grey and Scarlet: Letters From the War Areas by Army Sisters on Active Service* (London: Hodder and Stoughton, 1944), 46.
134 Sister TANS, 'Experiences of an Army Sister in the Middle East'.
135 Luker, 'Diaries from 1940–45' (24 December 1940).
136 Noakes, *Women in the British Army*, 6.
137 Bright, *Life in our Hands*, 5.
138 Iris Hooper, 'Life in a forward CCS', *Medical Gazette, 21 Army Group, Second Army* 1, 3 (June 1945) Wellcome Trust Collection, RAMC/1218/2/18, 51.
139 'Specialing' is the term used by nurses who are appointed to care for just one patient over a protracted period of time, usually because of a patient's serious physical or psychological illness.
140 Francie E. Brown, 'My dearest Win + Moll' (4 August 1944), IWM Documents 12472.
141 Hutchinson, 'My war and welcome to it', 36.
142 Pat Jalland, 'A culture of silent grief? The transformation of bereavement care in 20th century England', *Bereavement Care* 32, 1 (2013): 19.

2

Challenging nursing spaces

In June 1944, Sister Agnes Morgan wrote to her mother from a CCS near Rome:

> We are frightfully short staffed as a lot of the girls are working at forward F.D.S.s (field dressing stations) and we work like a C.C.S. except that we still think of ourselves as a Hospital and strive to do the 'little extra' that makes a difference between a C.C.S. and a Hospital! It is all impossible and rather hopeless, as the tide of human misery and suffering streams in too fast for us to do more than the bare necessities ... under canvas and all the water in a can, and all the sterilization by Primus stove![1]

The creation of spaces conducive to healing was a critical aspect of the provision of good nursing care. It had formed an important part of the advice given to women since Florence Nightingale. In *Notes on Nursing*, written just prior to the foundation of the Nightingale Training School at St Thomas' Hospital,[2] Nightingale directed her advice on how to care for the sickroom to the lady of the house.[3] In the 1906 edition of *Text-Book of Nursing*, Clara Weeks-Shaw maintained that 'The comfort and well-being of the invalid depend so great an extent upon his surroundings.'[4] According to Evelyn Pearce in her 1937 edition of *A General Textbook of Nursing*, 'A nurse with the gift of making her patients feel at home, and free from fear, inspires confidence and provides an atmosphere of peace, serenity and security which is so important an adjunct to the relaxation of mind and body necessary for recovery from disease.'[5] All these injunctions carry a twofold purpose: to provide comfort for the patient and to provide an environment that is physically 'healthful', to support healing. The nursing sisters of the British Army, having trained in the British hospital system, would have been well versed in the need to create and maintain and environment in which healing could take place. The zones into which they were posted during the Second World War and the spaces they were given in which to care for their patients were, however, rarely either favourable to health or to the 'serenity and security' needed for recovery.

In the previous chapter, fundamental nursing skills, so essential to all nurses, whether in a peacetime civilian hospital or on active service overseas, were considered. It argued that in order to care for sick and injured combatants, rituals of nursing care that had been so carefully nurtured in hospital training programmes and perfected as staff nurses, needed to be abandoned.[6] The nursing sisters of the British Army needed to 'humanise' their previously learnt nursing skills so as to manage the recovery of war-damaged men, and in doing so they needed to carefully broker a number of gender difficulties.

The purpose of this chapter is to examine the external challenges that nurses faced in working to pursue their healing skills. The chapter commences with an examination of the nature of home and the methods nurses employed to create a homely atmosphere in order to prepare physically able and psychologically stable men for battle. As I argue, Christmas celebrations were critical to this work. The chapter then considers the external forces that challenged all those concerned with the salvage of men in hospital units across the globe. Critical features of these challenges that are explored here are the weather and insect life. The final section examines the impact of the exigencies of war on the formation, organisation and clinical work of hospitals. Detailed focus will be given to the limited supplies of water for patient care and, finally, the effects of this and other external forces on the central work of surgery.

One of the common tropes often associated with the Second World War is that women made inroads into the world of masculine work such as engineering and then feminised that work.[7] Penny Summerfield's extensive studies on women's wartime work demonstrate a number of methods that were used to feminise men's work 'for the duration', sometimes by the employers to enable them to pay women less[8] and sometimes by the women themselves to retain their femininity, including the clothes they wore, hairstyles and make-up.[9] The pioneering use of women within the highly dangerous Special

Operations Executive (SOE) appears to suggest an inclusive attitude towards women's active participation in the war effort. However, being women not only influenced the work that they did as spies but also linked the efficacy of their espionage work to their femininity.[10] Allied female members of the SOE 'performed' as native French women, enabling them to move through German-controlled checkpoints to deliver secrets and equipment.[11] The dangerous work of espionage was made possible by the feminine form and traditional German attitudes that women's lives were located with 'Kinder, Kirche und Küche' (children, church and kitchen),[12] and not in the world of undercover activities.[13]

Whilst nursing was cast as feminine work, in the challenging environment of war it depended upon more masculine skills of innovation and ingenuity in order to manipulate the surroundings into habitable places. These skills link nursing judgements to ones that are high in 'indeterminacy', skills more usually associated with the critical clinical judgements of medicine,[14] and therefore requiring careful negotiation of professional and gender boundaries. In this way, the work of nurses on active service overseas reversed the more usual ideas about men and women's wartime work. Historians including Summerfield, Juliette Pattinson and Sonya O. Rose explore the feminisation of masculine work such as engineering and espionage. This chapter examines the manner in which British Army nurses 'masculinised' the very feminine work of home building.

'And HOME was miles away'

Sister C.M.S. Baker maintained that the troops fighting in the South-East Asian war, were 'not only fighting the Japanese but also the heat, disease and insects, and HOME was miles away'.[15] War weariness was felt by all, soldiers, nurses, doctors and orderlies alike. Although Morgan wrote of her homesickness in one of her earliest letters,[16] the effects of being away from home appear to have become harder the longer people were away: 'Tears trickled down our faces. Home!! ... We had been away from home for over two years, and it seemed like two centuries.'[17] Just two weeks before Sister Barbara Collins left her posting in Sierra Leone to get married, she wrote to her parents that despite the 'glamour of the tropics, there's no place like home'.[18] By

January 1945, Sister Mary Morris described a 'new element amongst our casualties this year – battle weariness. There is far less gaiety and Joie de Vivre. These men want to go home to their wives and families. They are tired after all the bloody battles of Normandy, Arnhem and Nijmegen.'[19]

The idea of home resonates throughout the testimonies, both as something to look forward to, and also as something to create in order to provide places for healing and recovery. Home is a significant place, as its ideology 'includes connotations of warmth, safety, emotional dependency'.[20] Penny Summerfield and Corinna Peniston-Bird argue that home is both a physical space and a metaphorical one, denoting the safety of home and the place of the nation.[21] Indeed, Summerfield maintains elsewhere that 'home' is the cornerstone of the nation.[22] Nationhood is imagined as an unchanging space in which 'we' are safe, safe because we are 'at home' – the place always imagined as providing the quintessence of 'emotional security'.[23]

For the troops on active service overseas the physical space of home was understood as a place of sanctity where they could experience 'a sense of belonging a feeling of relaxation and comfort'.[24] But it also needed to be a perennially secure space worthy of defending, a 'domestic idyll' that gave men something for which to continue fighting.[25] It was both home and the idea of home that kept the men going.[26] In creating a homelike space, nurses not only produced a place of parental safety, but one that embodied the 'homeland' – a utopian fantasy of the nation. This discourse supported the sick combatant's desire to return to the safety of the hearth and to preserve the likelihood of the hearth being as it was when he left, a 'British hearth'.[27] Creating spaces of domestic security was easier in base hospitals than in mobile units, but efforts were made to do so in every type of hospital unit. However, this was frequently stymied, not only by the environment but also by military decisions, including the frequent posting and reposting of hospital staff familiar to the combatant patients, as Sister P.M. Dyer experienced on Christmas Day 1944.[28]

Historians of twentieth-century war nursing have articulated the significance of home to soldier-patients. Creating a homelike space in the hospital ward or CCS was a critical method for encouraging men to believe they were closer to home and further from the horrors of trench and other forms of warfare. Many nurses recognised that 'this sense of safety promoted physical and emotional healing'.[29] Men needed to believe in home and have a space to heal after the horrors of war, and the female nurses believed that it was their role to provide it.[30] This gendered home-creation work was prevalent even into the latter half of the twentieth century. In the Vietnam war nurses argued that it was important for 'an American soldier to wake from surgery and see an American woman who symbolised home, safety and, an absence of war'.[31]

According to Jean Gilmour, 'nurses actively work to constitute hospitals as home places for patients'.[32] Yet this work created unforeseen complications within the status and positioning of female nurses on active service overseas. Crafting the domestic space was seen as lacking in complexity; indeed, as women's work it was understood as demanding neither skill nor strength, but dexterity and maternal qualities.[33] Margaret Higonnet and colleagues argue that war time may have 'impelled women out of the domestic sphere', but only to then maintain them in another place in which they were subordinate to men.[34] However, even for some key mid-twentieth-century 'feminists' the work of women within the home was not seen as denigrating but, rather, as their vital though different place in society to men's.[35] There is every suggestion that the Army nursing sisters of the Second World War saw this work in that way too.

However, the complexities of the position of nursing sisters on active service overseas were perhaps greater than the nurses themselves either wished or were able to admit. The reconstitution of hospital wards in a war zone to denote 'home' enabled female nurses to locate themselves in this most masculine of places without the need to 'ideologically' move beyond the family-oriented environment.[36] Nevertheless, by continuing to locate female nurses in a reimagined female space, it often prevented them from taking action outside of that situation. All other settings belonged to the masculine machine of war. On the ships that transported nurses and combatants to the various war zones, as officers in the British Army, the nurses had cabins and ate in the first-class dining room with the male officers, enjoying full officer status. The enlisted men, on the other hand, existed in steerage conditions in the bowels of the ships. Baker sailed from Glasgow to India in the spring of 1944. Once past the Bay of

Biscay, she and a colleague requested an inspection of the men in steerage, although why they did so is not clear:

> We were appalled (not a strong enough word) by the stench of sweat, sickness and socks in the sleeping quarters ... I am sure some men did not survive but we had no information about this, the contrast between the high living of officers and terrible low living of the men herded like cattle was terrible and we were shocked into silence. But what could we do? We did nothing.[37]

This lack of action on the part of the nursing staff is also shared in Sister Penny Salter's memoir, in which she recalled that the 'humidity and heat in the black-out conditions became appalling' as they cruised into the harbour at Freetown, Sierra Leone.[38] She continued, 'As for the troops, they were going berserk, for the state of affairs below deck had become almost suicidal, and only God knows how they survived those few desperate days and nights.'[39] Although both Salter and Baker show determination elsewhere in the personal testimonies of their wartime work, it was clear that there were boundaries to their influence that were non-negotiable.

Notwithstanding the political and social manoeuvrings to limit the power of nurses and potentially challenge the significance of their nursing role, most were aware of their importance in the salvage of men. They knew that on the ward they were the officer in charge and their work as creators of security for healing was vital to the war effort, a role that did not need further negotiation. Although, therefore, the homeliness of their work exemplified 'ordinariness' in nursing, it did not lessen its importance in the nurses' eyes. It is this very commonplaceness that can remind the patient of the 'essential nature of family',[40] and support recovery. Sister Mary Bond wrote:

> I became more and more used to working in the desert environment, although I missed many home comforts and I tried to make my patients feel as much at home as possible. One way I aimed to do this was to make their meals as enjoyable as I could ... The Australians and New Zealanders used to get parcels of food from home which they shared with other patients – these parcels came to be causes of celebration, particularly if there was a birthday to celebrate.[41]

Home was recreated in a number of ways, from the acquisition of pet dogs[42] to the creation of gardens. One TANS sister described the 'growing of trees and making of gardens around the wards and messes'.[43] Dorothy Bartlett described a matron who had soil shipped in so that she could create a garden.[44] The creation of gardens was seen as central to the recovery of those psychologically damaged by war, especially in such alien environments as that of a desert.[45] Sister Elsie Driver, posted to a 'Psychiatrical Neurological unit', wrote of the 'competition [that] was great between each ward, and one can well imagine what this meant, when all around stretched miles of desert'.[46] There were also more conventional techniques of creating a place for safety and recovery, methods that were bound in the traditional tripartite relationship between the father/doctor, mother/nurse and child/patient.[47] These practices included the naming of soldier-patients by nursing sisters and their medical officer colleagues as 'boys'.[48] Methods also included the celebration of patients' birthdays: 'A birthday party was going on round a bed in Sister Grace Thompson's ward. A group of sisters, doctors and orderlies were toasting the patient in lemonade. The patient, his chest swathed in bandages, was returning the toast in champagne.'[49]

The emblem of home was both a psychological creation and a physical one. Even making tea could provoke nostalgia for home.[50] Sister Ffolliott was proud to write to her Matron-in-Chief of their attempts to make the wards 'look nice, and when the beds were made up with the pretty blue blankets, in lieu of counterpanes, the effect was pleasing, and everyone admired them'.[51] In many ways, such attention to detail and aestheticism seems out of place in a war, but this nursing work was akin to the home-making work of wives and mothers and would therefore have served as important reminders of home. Some soldiers could not get used to domestic comforts. One sister wrote to the *Nursing Times* that her patients could not sleep in soft beds, preferring instead the hard floor.[52] However, nurses and the medical authorities more widely believed that it remained important to make the effort to cultivate homely environments. For those up-patients, attempts were made to bring cinema,[53] concerts and theatre into hospital complexes, and where these were not possible the Red Cross provided library books.[54] Sister Vera Jones maintained that 'The British "Tommy" does appreciate homely things',[55] and for Jones and others the perfect opportunity to provide this was at Christmas, a time when the thought is of others, especially for those so far from home.[56]

Christmas

War should not occur at Christmas. The 'extreme sentimentality about Christmas', coupled with the predominance of Christianity in both Germany and Britain in the First World War, gave rise to an 'acute sense of the incongruity of war on Christmas Day'.[57] The myths of the First World War Christmas truces are poignant, whether or not these actually occurred, because they remain the most vivid 'memories' of soldiers on both sides.[58] Arguably, because of the narratives of the Christmas truces in this earlier conflict, there is more focus on the impact of war on Christmas in writings on the First World War. However, the importance of this celebration as a link to home and tradition was understood as critical to maintaining morale.[59]

In a memorandum on 21 December 1939, the War Office stipulated that as far as possible Christmas Day and Boxing Day should be preserved as holidays on active service overseas.[60] Of that first Christmas at war, the diary for No.1 General Hospital stated that 'There have been no occasions of note over the Christmas period. Ways and means were found to provide suitable Christmas fare. Concerts and cine shows were given, and all the sub divisions of the hospital were very gaily and tastefully decorated.'[61] Yet sometimes the horrors of war did infiltrate the hoped-for Christmas spirit. There were intense difficulties in creating an atmosphere of joy when convoys of sick and injured men arrived, including those who had not slept in days and those without limbs from frostbite because no one had provided them with adequate uniform.[62] It is highly likely that amidst the hardship of war, the nursing sisters wanted to demonstrate their festive endeavours to the audiences of their correspondence and memoirs. Nevertheless, personal testimonies of all types, even private diaries, identify that despite the apparent impossibility of the situation at times, nurses took over the work of families, filling stockings, baking and developing Christmas cheer in war zones far from home.[63]

At Christmas 1940, Sister Jessie Wilson was working in a hospital in Greece when she wrote, 'We began to practice Christmas carols. Sisters decorated the hospital, preparations were in full swing for our first Christmas away from home, and everything was done to ensure that the boys had a good time.'[64] A year later she was posted to Helmieh in Egypt. Again she described the carol singing and Christmas dinner and the men joining in and helping with the decorations: 'One man thanked us for a wonderful day – his only regret was that his wife and children were not there to share the feast.'[65] Hearing of the invasion of Hong Kong made the memory of this Christmas hard. Her final Christmas was on a hospital ship in 1943 bound for Britain, and again the nursing staff sang, the men joined in and the wards were 'gay with decorations'.[66] Bartlett's recollections of Christmas 1943 in Kirkuk are equally as cheerful, with patients, sisters and officers alike enjoying the food, camaraderie and decorations.[67] Sister Underhill recalled the Christmases of 1940 and 1941, the first celebrated in Bethlehem and the second in Basra. Again, the nurses provided as much cheer and homeliness as was possible in a war.[68] Sister Catherine Butland even recalled the nurses wearing dresses and caps on Christmas day to cheer their patients with visions of womanliness whilst the men ate their Christmas dinner. After which there was a 'Fancy Dress football match at 3 p.m. Mobile Military Hospital versus Field Ambulance. Later we put on a concert party which was as much enjoyed by those taking part as by the audience.' Such joy was short lived as 'On Boxing Day we awoke at 4 a.m. to find the camp three foot under water.'[69] For those on Malta, the strafing began before Christmas 1941 and did not end until October 1942; their Christmas was not so joyous.[70] Despite nurses' attempts to make their soldier-patients' respite in hospital one that nurtured well-being, the external forces of war and weather frequently stymied such work.

'The winter was atrocious and in the summer very hot'

On her arrival in Europe in August 1943, Morgan wrote to her mother of the relief to be away from North Africa, 'no more whirling tantalising blowing sand …, with over all the dreadful brazen sun, glaring and roasting, until life became a bad dream'.[71] Poor weather conditions have been identified as having a significant effect on the health of soldiers and civilians in war zones. The conditions of war across the globe assaulted men's bodies and placed them under tremendous strain of disease and poor health. In the tropics men fell to malaria, bilharzia, heat exhaustion and heat stroke, whilst in the far north they developed 'frostbite, trench foot and snow-blindness'.[72] Historians of medicine and war in the twentieth century have considered the impact of poor weather on the troops. They have examined amongst other tragedies a typhus epidemic, caused by the inability to maintain personal hygiene in the trenches on the Eastern Front.[73] Joanna Bourke explores the legendary sub-zero temperatures at Stalingrad that led to the deaths of thousands of German troops from hypothermia and diseases associated with it.[74] Although there is an acknowledgement that poor weather led to disease, death and in some cases failure to win battles – poor weather hampered the movement of allied troops into Germany in the early months of 1945 – discussions of weather, apart from the profound difficulties it caused when attempting to evacuate men in torrential rain,[75] tend to be tangential to the actual medical care required or provided for the troops.[76]

The importance of the external environment to creating safe spaces in which successful nursing care can occur has meant that historians of war nursing offer more detailed narratives regarding weather conditions. However, most of these accounts have been focused on the First World War[77] – although, arguably, the weather and mud of the Western Front are, like the Christmas truces, part of the legend of the First World War. As Kirsty Harris maintains, 'Weather affected almost every aspect of nursing, significantly adding to the workload and forcing the nurses to change their usual processes.'[78] The mobility of the Second World War compared to that earlier global conflict did not give rise to the levels of 'trench-foot' caused by extensive periods in waterlogged trenches.[79] But poor weather conditions risked the development of other diseases. Men arrived at CCSs and hospitals debilitated due to the poor diets and dreadful weather conditions in which they had been living.[80] They were transported in open cattle-trucks in the pouring rain,[81] or in searing heat which led to severe burns,[82] and disembarked into the open air in snow.[83] Despite the protests of nurses at this treatment of both Allied and Axis troops, as these settings were outside the hospital wards, issues of gender, professional subordination and the exigencies of war prevented them from influencing more thoughtful care of the soldiers. This disregard for soldiers by some male officers may well have increased the nurses' determination to provide comfort once the men were in the hospital wards, spaces where nursing sisters were in charge. Sister Travis wrote in her report to Dame Katharine Jones:

> Our first cases were from neighbouring camps of [*sic*] straight off disembarking ships, the latter having an ambulance journey of two hours from the port to our hospital. Dysentery and malaria were the most common disease with, as the weather got colder, many cases of pneumonia and chest conditions aggravated by the sandy atmosphere.[84]

Travis continued that bread and hot soup were provided for their patients in the colder weather, and in hotter conditions, when possible, they tried to ensure that ice and fans were available in the wards. Nurses, doctors and orderlies may have been convinced of the vital role that the creation of a secure and comfortable environment played in the improved health of soldier-patients, but even in hospital, respite from the harsh weather conditions could be limited. Morgan wrote to her mother of the hospital in Italy that had previously been a POW camp, situated in a 'little hollow … The mountains are close in on us and most forbidding. It has rained unceasingly since our arrival, torrential down pours, with bitingly cold gusts blowing intermittently … However the day after we arrived our first convoy of 100 came in; and the next day another 100 and then next nearly 200.'[85] Not long after arriving to care for troops at the Anzio beachhead, an anonymous sister recalled the arrival of rain. After prolonged bitterly cold weather the ground was unable to cope with all the water, so the hospital flooded. With the battle continuing around them, the patients could not be evacuated and so their beds sunk deeper and deeper into the earth. 'Stretchers were raised on ration boxes, but the water still rose; hospital beds sank lower and lower until they were not much above ground level, and we waged a constant war attempting to keep patients, wards and bedding dry.'[86] One TANS sister wrote to Dame Katharine Jones of their particular problems in Iraq:

> This time the hospital was under canvas, and when we arrived the weather was bitterly cold, and this we felt very acutely, having come from a comparatively warm Palestine. It only rained for about three days in the part we were in, but as a result the whole country side was under water for at least 3 weeks, and for a long time the roads were quite impassable. The soil was clay and the water did not sink in.
>
> The hospital was about half a mile from the mess, and by the time we arrived on duty we were covered with mud, and hardly able to move with cold. The tents we worked in were not very waterproof, and when it rained we had to put buckets all the way down the middle of each tent,

> and ourselves [*sic*] had to wear storm caps, mackintoshes and Wellington boots, as well as any obtainable article of warm clothing. We worked under very 'active service' conditions, with one primus stove to heat everything for three tents, and a crude oil burner to heat the patients' washing water. There were crude oil heaters in each tent, which gave out a certain amount of warmth. At one time it was so cold that even the crude oil froze.[87]

Even without trying to combat disease and injury, managing the cold and rain, and the extreme fluctuations in temperature across the war zones of Europe and the Middle East, was a constant trial for nurses and patients alike and worked against the creation of homelike spaces: 'The winter was atrocious and in the summer very hot and glaring with innumerable storms.'[88] For those in the desert, it was the sandstorms that tested everyone's resolve. Underhill noted, 'we could never decide whether they were worse when they lashed our cold legs or when they covered us at a temperature of 127°F'.[89] One anonymous nursing sister wrote of the 'misfortune to spend October to April, the worst months from the point of view of desert weather, in this particular station [Geneifa]. Sandstorms left a film of sand over everything, no matter how carefully they were guarded against. These sandstorms alternated with rainstorms.'[90] Sister D.S. Low described the changes in the weather from blinding heat to sandstorms and deluges of rain.[91]

The weather in all war zones had a considerable effect on the nurses and their patients. But it was also the ramifications of the weather conditions that significantly hampered the effectiveness of the nurse–patient encounter. Men expected their nurses to be kind and provide bodily comforts for them.[92] But the freezing night temperatures in tented wards, rainfall that flooded whole hospitals and the insects that abounded in hot and dusty climes meant that whilst the nursing sisters wanted to ease the trials of war, such comforts were not always possible. Of course, not all nurses were able to drop their long-learned routines and ideas about good nursing and a disciplined hospital ward. The matron of a group of newly arrived nursing sisters in Tobruk was appalled to view filthy blankets hanging in the doorways of the wards and demanded that the orderlies remove these 'ripe' drapes. The disgruntled orderlies who had up till then been running the ward did remove them, but only under duress, understandably annoyed at being placed under the authority of a female nurse who had little comprehension of desert conditions. Soon after the offending articles were removed a sandstorm blew uninhibited through the wards; the blankets went back up.[93]

'Out came the beasties'

When Salter arrived at Ramree Island off the coast of Burma, the advent of convoys of casualties from Rangoon and Elephant Point coincided with the monsoon season: 'it rained and it rained and it rained – the monsoon arrived with a vengeance. With the rains, out came the beasties – flying ants, bats and mosquitoes in their droves.'[94] All the nursing sisters in the Second World War complained about the mosquitoes and flies, as had their predecessors in the First World War.[95] The flies were everywhere, 'in their thousands',[96] bringing distress and disease to their patients, their colleagues and themselves and making nursing care a considerable challenge. Penny Starns argues that flies in the desert war zone actually improved healing because of the maggots that they produced,[97] but mostly they were considered to be vectors of disease.[98] Morgan wrote to her mother, 'remember that men with helpless arms cannot keep the flies at bay!'[99] This inability would have a considerable effect on the men and their health, given that flies were a source of infection as they bred dysentery and infiltrated wounds and caused sepsis.[100] As one sister in the desert maintained, 'The campaign against flies was fought quite as much a part of the war as any tank battle, brainy attractive posters were placed in convenient places. Patients and personnel were all made "fly conscious". Fly netting over the doors and windows. Refuse was not allowed to accumulate.'[101] Fly netting was crucial, as without it, 'the wards were black with them [flies]'.[102] But it was not only flies which were a constant annoyance to patients, ants too were a significant problem:

> I had had a very busy night, and was preparing to go off duty when a patient called me and said that there were 'things' crawling all over his badly burned leg. On investigation I found almost a complete ants' nest in the bed! The ants, one of the very small brown kind, had come in the ward window, and climbed up the patient's Balkan beam, and got into his bed, in spite of the fact that the legs of the beam had been well saturated with paraffin the day before. It took me nearly three quarters of an hour to remove every ant and to redress the leg, and I thought I had learnt my lesson and would see that

> such a thing did not occur again. However, it happened a few mornings later when a sailor with a horribly burnt face, which was completely brown with Tannic Acid, called and said that here seemed to be 'things' crawling on his face. After close examination to my horror I found ants all over his face and hand, and even in his ears. Apparently he had moved his locker so that it was touching his bed, and the little beasts had got in that way.[103]

The nursing sisters' attempts to ensure their patients were safe and comfortable were severely hampered by the external conditions of weather and wildlife. However, it was not only the natural environment that worked against the creation of homelike spaces. The war itself, which assaulted supply lines, bombed buildings and damaged electricity, water and sanitary systems, also played a part in stymying the nurses' desire to make hospital wards secure and homely places for healing.

'Something thrilling in the shaping of a new hospital'

Personal testimonies from Army nursing sisters identify concerns over their ability to ensure that hospital wards were as safe and comfortable a place for their soldier-patients as possible. Included in these were specific worries about the lack of water, limited equipment, especially for sterilising surgical instruments, and primitive sanitation in all war zones. There were more general concerns too over the physical spaces in which their patients were to be treated. Hutted wards were more secure places for patient care, more comfortable and easier to keep sand free. However, it was not unknown for them to become infested with bugs, at which point they needed to be demolished.[104] The purpose of mobile units was to admit, triage and evacuate all but the most seriously ill and injured within 24 hours. Tented hospitals were ideal therefore, as they could be set up within hours and expanded as more convoys arrived. Given their role, they required little furniture and minimal comforts, thus making their establishment and dismantling even faster.[105] However, in poor weather conditions they frequently became water-logged, or blew away.[106] Military medical authorities and hospital staff therefore negotiated the fine line of expediency between mobile units that were essential to providing early treatment intervention, but that were subject to the vagaries of the weather, or more comfortable hospitals in which patients could recover, but that took several months to build and could easily become the object of an infestation.

By 1944 and the Second Front, the creation of a tented hospital from scratch was a well-orchestrated event. The formation of a human force that was so well rehearsed that it could organise itself in the harshest of environments was an essential part of creating a successful army. Civilian men were turned into soldiers through 'highly ritualised' training to create a cohesive unit that could respond almost automatically to commands.[107] Whilst early in the war, nurses like Sister Mary Bond had learnt their Army skills on service in the deserts of North Africa and the Middle East, the need for nurses and orderlies to be trained in Britain before leaving for active service overseas soon became apparent.[108] Importantly, this meant that on arriving at a suitable site, personnel were able to establish a full working hospital within three months and a mobile unit in a matter of hours.[109] Nurses were trained to label and pack instruments so that they could be located as soon as a unit found a suitable place for a hospital to be situated.[110] Sometimes, the rapidity of convoys was such that tents needed to be erected around the patients as they arrived. In a report to Dame Katharine Jones, one sister, attached to 10th CCS, which accepted casualties from the Battle of El Alamein,[111] wrote:

> Only fifty beds are allowed to a C.C.S. the rest of the patients are nursed on the stretchers on which they are brought in. These stretchers were packed side by side on either side of the wards and then others were put head to foot down the centre, this left a narrow passage way about a foot wide each side. A spare tent materialised from some unknown source and was used to extend the Officers' ward, it was literally put up around the patients, the patients were there first.[112]

If a unit was fortunate, a building could be requisitioned for use as a hospital. Some, like schools with their large open rooms, were ideal. Other types of buildings, especially hotels, created difficulties for nurses as patients were in single rooms and therefore could not be seen at all times.[113] Some were clean and others rat infested, but at least they had walls.[114] There were times when it was possible to take over an actual hospital, although these had frequently been shelled. Arriving in Tobruk after the evacuation of the Italians, a sister wrote that the hospital was 'little more than a ruin, for all it was waterproof and everything clean'. The organisation of the hospital was greatly supported by the apparent rapidity of the Italian evacuation, which meant that much of their supplies and equipment, including dressings, had been left behind, enabling the efficient admission and treatment of patients.[115]

Sister Winifred Mountford's experiences in Brittany with the British Expeditionary Force (BEF) in January 1940 were of setting up hospitals in schools, closing them up, moving on and setting up a new one. They initially set up No. 8 General Hospital in Brest with only oil heaters for warmth, and she recalled quickly learning to 'improvise in every way whilst nursing under these conditions'. By March 1940 the hospital was moved to another school, this time in Rennes, by which time the fighting had started in earnest and the wounded began to arrive, 'the ward was full of beds and many times stretchers on the floor too'.[116] Sister Ffolliott thought there was 'something thrilling in the shaping of a new hospital, and in seeing uninteresting-looking huts acquire character and evolve into wards'.[117] Sister Allen wrote to Dame Katharine of the ingenious bulldozing of the desert to create an airstrip for the transportation of blood and critically ill patients.[118] If Underhill was impressed when her desert 'cantonment' was built in just six months, she was even more so when the operating theatre was rigged with emergency lighting, 'arranged by the "finding" of a derelict steam-roller that was later discovered to have lost its engine'.[119] This irreverent procuring of wreckage and old equipment to manufacture into utensils proved essential in the creation of hospitals. It also provided valuable occupational therapy to support the rehabilitation of the sick and essential furniture for the hospital wards, developing them into homely environments:

> One of the bed patients, feeling the lack of anywhere to put his photographs, instructed the walking cases to go out and procure from the transport section as many of the old type of petrol tins as they could. These he proceeded to cut (to the great detriment of the plaster shears) and flatten out. This done the edges were hammered under, the narrow ends turned one each over a bedstead and a shelf formed. These shelves were of great value to the patients and were also appreciated by the nursing staff.[120]

Indeed, when no such equipment was available, the ability of hospitals to function could be quite limiting. Writing to the *Nursing*

Times, one nursing sister did not so much bemoan the lack of new primus stoves whilst on Malta in 1941 and 1942, but the lack of parts to mend old ones.[121] The nurses' testimonies suggest that they were proud to be in active service conditions,[122] and Ffolliott was clearly pleased that the staff in her West African hospital were 'masters of improvisation'.[123] It was, however, in accessing water across the Middle East and Africa that the nursing sisters' capacity for creativity was to be most substantially tested. Despite the criticality of water to a nurse's work, their capacity to reuse and recycle and still maintain patient safety demonstrates their ingenuity in the face of the indeterminate.

'Much trouble with our water supply'

Acknowledging that nursing on active service overseas had some particular 'trials and tribulations',[124] one of the most all-encompassing of these in maintaining both personal hygiene and the nurses' abilities to heal their combatant patients was the lack of water in hospitals across Africa and the Middle East. Jones wrote to her parents from No. 60 General Hospital in Egypt in August 1941: 'It is very hot and oppressive here, and will be for the next two months at least. We are having much trouble with our water supply and are rationed quite severely where water is concerned.'[125] Low was posted to the 32 General Hospital near Khartoum: 'Water is brought by road from a distance by Diesel lorries holding thousands of gallons of water, but when these break down, which happens fairly frequently, water is sent in small tanks by night and day services to replenish our huge cisterns, but the supply is quite insufficient for our needs.'[126] According to Sister Betty Parkin, the lack of water made barrier nursing 'very consuming of time and energy with water taps and soakways outside'.[127] After the battle for El Alamein in the autumn of 1942, the damage to drains in Tripoli and the limited fuel supplies added to the problems, as it was difficult to transport sufficient uncontaminated water.[128]

The paucity of water meant that patients and staff would be rationed with their drinking water, and also water for cooking, cleaning, laundry and patient hygiene.[129] Allen wrote of the 'brackish' water that was used to make cups of tea.[130] Sister Joyce Hilder wrote to the *Nursing Times* in 1942 informing its readers of the water shortages in Sierra Leone, a country in which the humidity in the

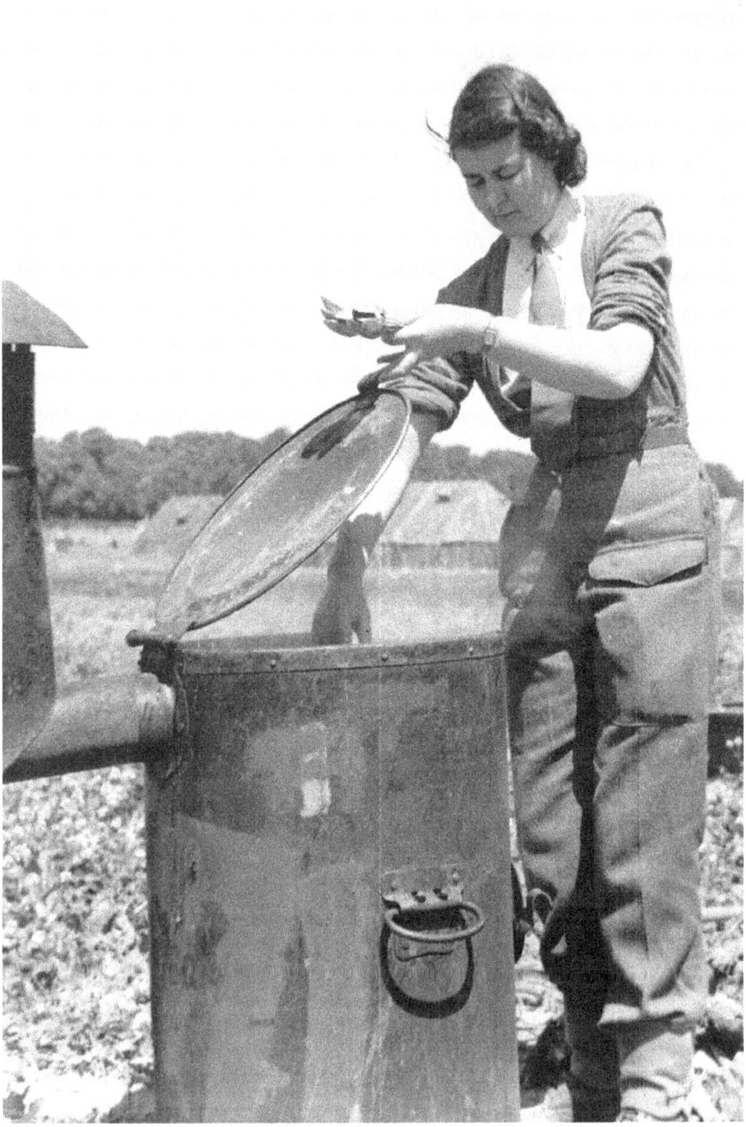

4 Sister Pamela Bright getting hot water from a Sawyer stove at 88 General Hospital, La Deliverande. Hospital facilities on active service were frequently situated outside, rather than in the hospital building. This significantly added to the nurses' work.

rainy season was unbearable. Between January and May, however, the shortage was such that they could use water for only three hours a day, '6.30–7.30am, 12.30–1.30pm, 5.30–6.30pm. There was no hot water and gas at all.'[131] Yet, despite these considerable challenges, nurses appear to have been able to improvise and provide a reasonable level of care: 'All water for washing patients, washing crockery and other general purposes had to be heated on primus stoves but we seemed to manage. All water for drinking purposes had to be chlorinated and fetched from a 500 gallon tank in tins.'[132]

If nurses across Africa and the Middle East struggled to ensure patient comfort with only limited supplies of water, of critical concern to the medical services in general was the lack of water for surgery. Even if there was water, limited equipment for sterilising instruments, lack of time or of electricity could challenge even the most experienced of teams.

'We had no pause for clearing during cases'

The organisation of front-line surgery was predicated on injured men receiving their initial treatment within eight hours, and then the next interval for treatment was to be no more than ten days. The wounds of the Second World War were multiple and complex, caused by increasingly technological and mobile machines that bombarded soldiers with shells, grenades and mines, wounds that tore away flesh, muscle and limbs and left gaping holes where abdominal tissue had once been.[133] The need for primary excision of wounds within twelve hours in order for success to be anticipated meant surgical teams needed to be mobile and forward. An immobile CCS could not be sent to the casualty, so the surgeon and therefore the surgical team needed to be sent to the casualty.[134] However, surgery in front-line war zones lacked even basic amenities, including electricity and running water. If there was water but no electricity, primus stoves were used to sterilise instruments. Paraffin lamps were used to illuminate the operating theatre, although these lamps did not provide sufficient light for the operations.[135] When there was a lack of water Lysol and carbolic acid were used to sterilise instruments.

The haunting writings of the surgical teams,[136] with ever-present pain and the ethical dilemmas of war surgery,[137] pervade medical histories of war. The historiography of the Second World War includes improvements in orthopaedic and blood transfusion technologies.[138] Historians of war nursing explore the practicalities of surgical work, including those aspects that are related to the patients themselves, wound care, asepsis and pain relief.[139] Surgical work needs sterility in order to ensure patient safety. Yet, despite the difficulties presented in forward areas in providing a sterile environment and instruments, this aspect of war surgery has been largely excluded from the historical canon. Although the difficulties of sanitation may have been the most severe in mobile units that needed to move rapidly into battle zones to provide early treatments, most hospitals in overseas theatres of war experienced poor sanitation and provision of clean water. This, coupled with limited access to electricity in some areas, led to significant problems in the sterilisation of surgical instruments, a long-standing and critical role for the theatre sister.

According to Evelyn Pearce's 1937 edition of *A General Textbook of Nursing*, instruments should be boiled for 20 minutes in a steriliser with a closed lid containing 1% sodium bicarbonate.[140] The lack of time, electricity, sterilisers and water meant that such practices in a war zone were curtailed considerably. Sister Mogg described the constant attention that was required to the primus stoves, sometimes the most advanced technology available for sterilising equipment. In the absence of sufficient water and fuel, it was essential that these did not fail during a 'rush'. One orderly's time was completely occupied pumping the stoves 'in order to maintain sufficient heat for sterilising the drums; and keep the instruments boiling. The use of stoves, together with the inevitable sand blowing about unavoidably caused a lot of dirt.'[141] Sister L'Estrainge also described the difficulties with primus stoves and the necessity to have an orderly constantly in charge of them.[142] In the theatre where Sister Pam Dunnett worked, so close to the front line that the surgical team could barely hear each other over the noise of the shelling, all the sterilising was done in a fish kettle.[143] Memories such as Dunnett's that recall the amusing and bizarre aspects of war service are probably filtered through what Lynn Abrams calls 'flash-bulb' memory.[144] The image of a fish kettle being used for sterilising fits with recollections of personal importance as nurses engaged in increasingly novel ways to manage their soldier-patients' care in hostile environments. The emotional significance of such memories does not mean that they are less factual. Dunnett's is not the only testimony that remembered the use of odd utensils for sterilising. Thus, even flash-bulb memories, usually associated with feelings and vivid experiences, can provide the reader with a real sense of the lives of nurses on active service overseas.

Dyer wrote of the great difference in running a surgical ward in England as compared to West Africa where there were 'No electric switches to switch on for sterilisation of the towels and instruments, the alternative being wood fires to boil all our requirements, and sterility being carried out as well as possible.'[145] In 1945, Dyer was posted to Comilla, where the process for managing surgical interventions was no more sophisticated: 'Our medical and surgical equipment was of the barest necessity, and our sterilisation was prepared in a billy can over a wood fire or else by flaming the bowls with methylated spirits. Primitive means but it was surprising how efficiently all these arduous toils were carried out.'[146] Inevitably, as Dyer identified, sometimes there was no water for sterilising surgical equipment and alternatives had to be found. Sister L'Estrainge wrote that surgical instruments would be immersed in carbolic acid and then rinsed, although she states that this was done only on the orders of a naval surgical specialist.[147] These improvisations suggest that nurses willingly worked with their medical colleagues in subverting their long-held ritualised procedures.

Butland, of No. 5 General Hospital with the BEF in France between 1939 and the spring of 1940, was ordered to join the 159 Field Ambulance of the RAMC in a hamlet outside Tournai. This order was in itself unusual, as normally, Butland's memoir informed its readers, 'there are *no* Sisters on the staff of a Field Ambulance'.

> We worked in the theatre continuously for over 12 hours, having one short break of about ½ hour when we ran out of anaesthetics. During break we managed to make a cup of tea. Our sterile dressings were soon used up and we improvised by soaking the uncut rolls of gauze in a Lysol solution and cutting off a length as needed. It was impossible to keep track of the patients operated on. Every man needing surgical attention was brought to the theatre. We had no pause for clearing during cases. As one man was removed from the operating table another was placed on it. Instruments were hurriedly washed and then flung into a bowl containing pure Lysol. We kept on the same pair of rubber gloves until they split, just scrubbing them in pure Lysol and washing them off under the tap. The whole day the hamlet was being machine gunned from the air. What we had taken to be

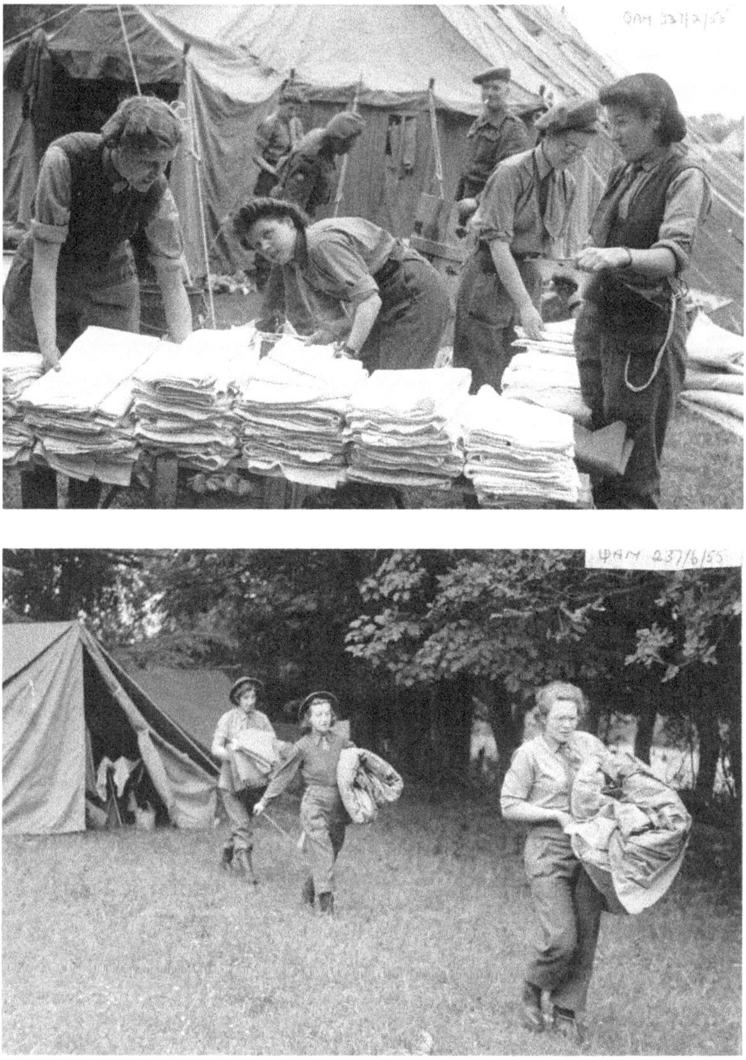

5 Normandy, 1944. Preparing the beds … When nurses were posted into war zones, like their male soldier colleagues, they needed to prepare themselves for the possibility of shelling.

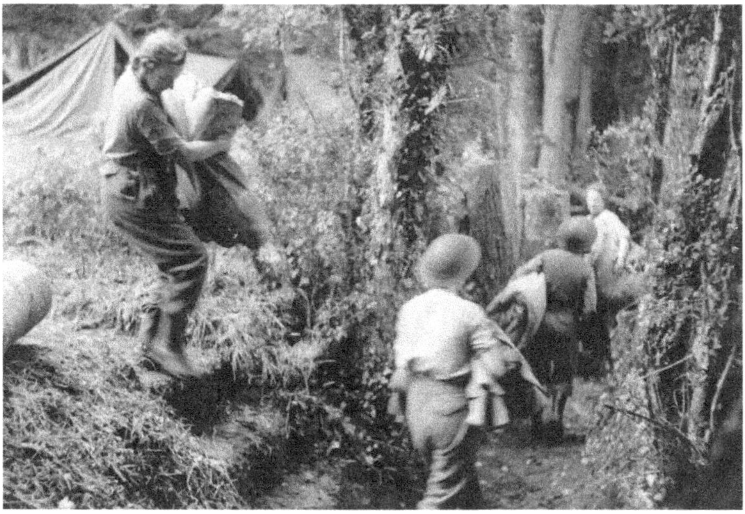

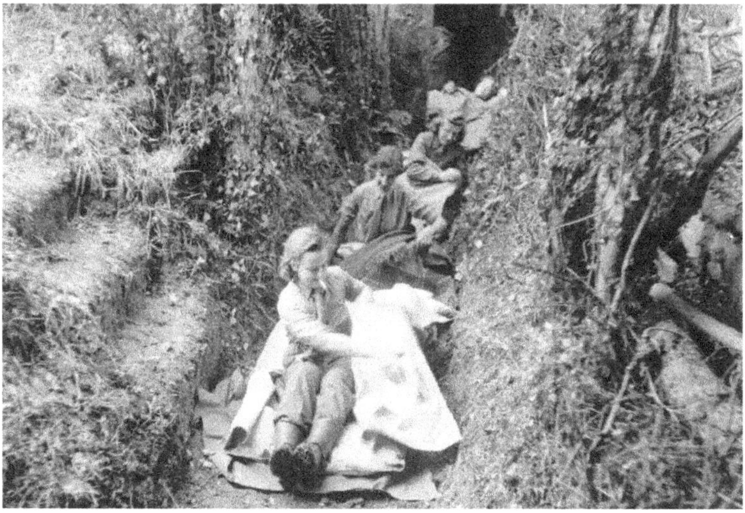

> the continuous 'blowing' of the methylated spirit sterilizers, was actually the school being attacked.[148]

Although nursing sisters were not always part of these forward teams, their presence became more prevalent as the war progressed and the improvements in patient care were acknowledged. Santanu Das' First World War nurses were witnesses to the war, a status that 'suggests a certain degree of exteriority and detachment'.[149] Their range of engagement in all war zones and front-line duty suggest that in the Second World War nurses were not witnesses but central players. The sheer volume of men who needed care in the Second World War impacted on surgical practice and, ultimately, the place of nurses. In previous wars female nurses had been posted into dangerous environments, but rarely had such a critical mass of women been required to care for patients under fire so close to the front line. However, placing women so close to the danger of the front line subverted the nostalgia of home, it placed women in men's space. Furthermore, there were fears in some quarters that by facing the challenges of war service, women became 'hardened'.[150] Nevertheless, the medical military authorities realised that they needed trained female nurses in the most challenging of war zones to salvage men for battle. This realisation may have won over gender sensibilities but, as will be discussed in the next chapter, it did not mean that the presence of women in hostile front-line duty was unproblematic.

Conclusion

British nursing sisters on active service overseas faced a number of significant external challenges to providing the nursing that they believed was required to recover men. Extreme weather conditions, limited water supplies, equipment and electricity combined to hinder all aspects of patient care. The often hostile places in which nurses worked demanded that they develop clinical skills and the ability to improvise and innovate in order create healing spaces for their soldier-patients. However, it was the highly feminised home-maker work that created these spaces, which the nurses themselves credited to be an essential aspect of the healing process in which they were the critical performers.

There were nevertheless a number of complexities inherent in nurses' crafting themselves as professionals who established feminine spaces in a masculine environment. These ideas perpetuated the accepted wisdom about the proper role of nurses as women. As female nurses, their gender and professional status meant that they were powerless to help the troops outside the circumscribed arena of the hospital. They may have been officers in charge of the wards, but outside that domain their influence was severely curtailed by the male military and medical machine. The next chapter explores the contradictions that nurses' 'femaleness' created on active service overseas. It will be argued that as women, they were subject to a more heightened scrutiny than their male colleagues. However, as the only women officers in war zones, they were encouraged to take on privileges and freedoms that they would not have experienced on home soil.

Notes

1 Agnes Kathleen Dunbar Morgan, 'Still with the lamp: Letters to my mother by an Army Nursing Sister. Egypt – North Africa – Sicily – Italy, 1941–1944', letter 84 (July 1944), CMF near Rome, Imperial War Museum Private Papers (hereafter IWM) Documents 16686.
2 For detailed discussion on the reform of the occupation of nursing see for example, Robert Dingwall, Anne Marie Rafferty and Charles Webster, *An Introduction to the Social History of Nursing* (London: Routledge, 1988); Monica E. Baly, *Nursing and Social Change* (London: Routledge, 1995); Anne Marie Rafferty, *The Politics of Nursing Knowledge* (London: Routledge, 1996).
3 Florence Nightingale, *Notes on Nursing: What It Is and What It Is Not* (New York: Dover Publications, 1969).
4 Clara Weeks-Shaw, *A Text-Book of Nursing: For the Use of Training Schools, Families and Private Students* (3rd edn) (New York: D. Appleton and Company, 1906), 14.
5 Evelyn Pearce, *A General Textbook of Nursing: A Comprehensive Guide to the Final State Examinations* (London: Faber and Faber, 1937), 2.
6 Cynthia Toman, *An Officer and a Lady: Canadian Military Nursing and the Second World War* (Vancouver: University of British Columbia Press, 2007), 138.
7 Susan R. Grayzel, *At Home and Under Fire: Air Raids and Culture in Britain from the Great War to the Blitz* (Cambridge: Cambridge University Press, 2012).
8 Penny Summerfield, 'What women learned from the Second World War',

History of Education 18, 3 (1989): 214; Penny Summerfield, *Reconstructing Women's Wartime Lives: Discourse and Subjectivity in Oral Histories of the Second World War* (Manchester: Manchester University Press, 1998), 126–38.

9 Summerfield, *Reconstructing Women's Wartime Lives*, 91.

10 Juliette Pattinson, *Behind Enemy Lines: Gender, Passing and the Special Operations Executive in the Second World War* (Manchester: Manchester University Press, 2007), 136.

11 Pattinson argues that one of the critical recruitment strategies was that members of the SOE had to speak French as a French native, not the fluent French of a foreigner. Many members of the SOE had lived in France for extended periods, or attended school in France. Pattinson, *Behind Enemy Lines*, 32–7.

12 Pattinson, *Behind Enemy Lines*, 139.

13 Pattinson, *Behind Enemy Lines*, see particularly Chapter 6: '"The best disguise": Performing femininities'.

14 Michael Traynor, Maggie Boland and Niels Buus, 'Autonomy, evidence and intuition: Nurses and decision-making', *Journal of Advanced Nursing* 66, 7 (2010): 1584–91.

15 C.M.S. Baker, 'Aftermath of war, September 1945', IWM Documents 6341, 14. 'HOME' in upper case in the original.

16 Morgan, 'Still with the lamp', letter 9 (November 1941), MEF, 2.

17 Jessie Sarah Catherine Wilson, 'We also served, 1940 …', 33, UK Centre for the History of Nursing (UKCHN) Archive, University of Manchester.

18 Barbara Collins, 'My dearest Mummy and Daddy' (10 May 1941), 5, 'Letters home from Sierra Leone', 1940–1941, UKCHN Archive, University of Manchester.

19 Mary Morris, 'The diary of a wartime nurse' (23 January 1945), 169, IWM Documents 4850; Mary Morris, *A Very Private Diary: A Nurse in Wartime*, ed. Carol Acton (London: Weidenfeld and Nicolson, 2014), 147.

20 David Benjamin, 'Afterword', *The Home: Words, Interpretations, Meanings and Environments* (Aldershot: Ashgate, 1995) 294. See also Jeanne Moore, '"Placing the home in context', *Journal of Environmental Psychology* 20 (2000): 207–17.

21 Penny Summerfield and Corinna Peniston-Bird, 'Women in the firing-line: The Home Guard and the defence of gender boundaries in Britain in the Second World War', *Women's History Review* 9, 2 (2000): 232.

22 Penny Summerfield, 'Gender and war in the twentieth century', *The International History Review* 19, 1 (1997): 6.

23 Sonya O. Rose, *Which People's War? National Identity and Citizenship in Britain, 1939–1945* (Oxford: Oxford University Press, 2003, Kindle edition), loc. 323–347.

24 Judith Sixsmith, 'The meaning of home: An exploratory study of

environmental experience', *Journal of Environmental Psychology* 6 (1986): 294.

25 Lucy Noakes, '"Serve to save": Gender, citizenship and Civil Defence in Britain, 1937–41', *Journal of Contemporary History* 47, 4 (2012):736.

26 Susan R. Grayzel, '"Fighting for the idea of home life": *Mrs Miniver* and Anglo-American representations of domestic morale', in Philippa Levine and Susan R. Grayzel (eds), *Gender, Labour, War and Empire* (London: Palgrave Macmillan, 2009), 145.

27 Rose, *Which People's War?*, loc. 339.

28 P.M. Dyer, 'When life was grey and scarlet: A recollection of life as an Army Nursing Sister', 63, Museum of Military Medical (hereafter MMM) QARANC/PE/1/151/DYER Box 8.

29 Christine E. Hallett, *Containing Trauma: Nursing Work in the First World War* (Manchester: Manchester University Press, 2009), 178.

30 Kirsty Harris, *More than Bombs and Bandages: Australian Army Nurses at Work in World War I* (Newport: Big Sky Publishing, 2011, Kindle edition), loc. 2294; Cynthia Toman, *Sister Soldiers of the Great War: The Nurses of the Canadian Army Medical Corps* (Vancouver: University of British Columbia Press, 2016), 34.

31 Kara Dixon Vuic, *Officer, Nurse, Woman: The Army Nurse Corps in the Vietnam War* (Baltimore, MD: Johns Hopkins University Press, 2010, Kindle edition), loc. 139.

32 Jean A. Gilmour, 'Hybrid space: Constituting the hospitals as a home space for patients', *Nursing Inquiry* 13, 1 (2006): 18.

33 Penny Summerfield, '"They didn't want women back in that job": The Second World War and the construction of gendered work histories', *Labour History Review* 63, 1 (1998): 86.

34 Margaret Randolph Higonnet, Jane Jenson, Sonya Michel and Margaret Collins Weitz, 'Introduction', in Margaret Randolph Higonnet, Jane Jenson, Sonya Michel and Margaret Collins Weitz (eds), *Behind the Lines: Gender and the Two World Wars* (New Haven, CT: Yale University Press, 1987), 3.

35 Caitriona Beaumont, 'Citizens not feminists: The boundary negotiated between citizenship and feminism by mainstream women's organisations in England, 1928–39', *Women's History Review* 9, 2 (2000): 411–29; Caitriona Beaumont, 'The women's movement, politics and citizenship, 1918–1950s', in Ina Zweiniger-Bargielowska (ed.), *Women in Twentieth-Century Britain* (Harlow: Pearson Education, 2001); Barbara Caine, *English Feminism, 1780–1980* (Oxford: Oxford University Press, 2001); Maria DiCenzo, '"Our Freedom and its Results": Measuring progress in the aftermath of suffrage', *Women's History Review* 23, 3 (2014): 421–40.

36 For a brief discussion of the preservation of 'the male/female, public/private dichotomy' in the Second World War, see Lucy Noakes, *War and the*

British: Gender, Memory and National Identity (London: I.B. Tauris, 1998), 50.

37 Baker, 'Aftermath of war, September 1945: A view of war by an officer of the QAIMNS (October 1943 to May 1945), 8.

38 Penny Salter, 'Long ago and far away: A distant memory': A diary, c. 1938–1970, 52, UKCHN Archive, University of Manchester and IWM Documents 17649.

39 Salter, 'Long ago and far away', 53.

40 Beverley Taylor, 'Ordinariness in nursing as therapy', in Richard McMahon and Alan Pearson, *Nursing as Therapy* (2nd edn) (Cheltenham: Stanley Thornes, 1998), 70.

41 Mary Bond, *Wartime Experiences from the Midnight Sun to Belsen* (Cardigan: E.L. Jones and Son, 1994), 30.

42 Catherine M. Butland, 'Sisters in battledress or the chosen few or follow fate', 56, MMM QARANC/PE/1/74/BUTL, Box 8.

43 Sister TANS, 'Desert hospital, 1941 and 1942', in Ada Harrison (ed.), *Grey and Scarlet: Letters from the War Areas by Army Sisters on Active Service* (London: Hodder and Stoughton, 1944), 118.

44 Dorothy Bartlett, *Nurse in War* (London: P.R. Macmillan, 1961), 83.

45 According to Edgar Jones and Simon Wessely, the percentages of psychiatric disorders were much higher for the desert war than previously thought. Edgar Jones and Simon Wessely, 'Psychiatric battle casualties: An intra- and interwar comparison', *The British Journal of Psychiatry* 178 (2001): 242–7.

46 Elsie Driver, 'Dear Miss Soutar' (9 July 1944), MMM QARANC uncatalogued archive.

47 Sue Hawkins, *Nursing and Women's Labour in the Nineteenth Century: The Quest for Independence* (London: Routledge, 2010), 22.

48 Morgan repeatedly refers to her patients as 'boys' within her letters to her mother. This not only enabled her and her colleagues to engage in intimate care without raising the spectre of sex in their work, but also to hide such possibilities from family back home. See, for example, 'Boys that we'd nursed months ago popped in from surrounding Camps', letter 25 (April 1942), MEF, 1–2; 'I wish that you could just see "my boys" for one minute. You wouldn't want me to leave them', letter 55 (July 1943), MEF, 2; 'my boys mean so much to me', letter 61 (September 1943), CMF, 3; 'both Navy boys and absolute dears', letter 65 (October 1943), CMF, 1. Morgan, 'Still with the lamp'; Catherine Hutchinson recalled a tropical diseases specialist who rarely addressed the patients by rank, 'but by Christian name or "my boy"'. Catherine Arnold Hutchinson, 'My war and welcome to it', Memoir, 110, IWM Documents 11950.

49 Jean Bowden, *Grey Touched with Scarlet: The War Experiences of Army Nursing Sisters* (London: Robert Hale, 1959), 146–7.

50 Emma Newlands, *Civilians into Soldiers: War, the Body and British*

Army Recruits, 1939–45 (Manchester: Manchester University Press, 2014), 163.

51 L.R. Ffolliott, 'Account of work and experience in West Africa, May 1941–June 1943', MMM QARANC/CF/4/5/9/WW2, box 68.

52 Anonymous, 'In step with the QAs 8. – Hospital ship (Part I) *Nursing Times* (30 September 1944): 678.

53 D.S. Low, 'Sudan: 32 General Hospital in the Middle East 1939–1942' and 'Sudan and Eritrea, 1939–1942' (May 1942) MMM QARANC/PE/1/319/WW2 box 68; Jane L. Forrest, 'Dear madam' (20 April 1943), MMM QARANCPE/297/Jones collections and accounts 1943, box 68.

54 Hutchinson, 'My war and welcome to it', 38.

55 Vera Jones, 'My dear mother and father' (26 May 1944), *A Time To Remember: A Record of Nursing Experiences, Impressions and Travels During World War II Contained in Letters Sent Home from The East* (London: Athena Press, 2005), 274.

56 Julia Brock, Jennifer W. Dickey, Richard J.W. Harker and Catherine M. Lewis (eds), *Beyond Rosie: A Documentary History of Women and World War II* (Fayetteville, AK: University of Arkansas Press, 2015, Kindle edition), loc. 2316.

57 John Terraine, 'Christmas 1914, and after', *History Today* 29 (1979): 781.

58 Iain Adams, 'A game for Christmas? The Argylls, Saxons and football on the Western Front, December 1914', *The International Journal of the History of Sport* 32, 11–12 (2015): 1395–415.

59 There is little written on this as part of the British attitude, but see, for example, William R. Brown, 'The American girl and the Christmas tree: World War II soldier poets look at what the G.I.s were fighting for', *Journal of American Culture* 8, 2 (1985): 25–30.

60 No.1 General Hospital, 'Memorandum. 4. Routine, Christmas and Boxing Day (21 December 1939), TNA WO 177/1091.

61 No.1 General Hospital, 'Diary' (26 December 1939), TNA WO 177/1091.

62 Agnes Barnett, 'Working with allies', in Barbara Mortimer (ed.), *Sisters: Extraordinary True-Life Stories from Nurses in World War Two* (London: Hutchinson, 2012), 174.

63 Harris, *More than Bombs and Bandages*, loc. 2402.

64 Wilson, 'We also served, 1940 …', 12.

65 Wilson, 'We also served, 1940 …', 29.

66 Wilson, 'We also served, 1940 …'.

67 Bartlett, *Nurse in War*, 111.

68 D. Underhill, 'To the Matron-in-Chief, Q.A.I.M.N.S., Dear Dame Katherine [*sic*]', MMM QARANC uncatalogued archive.

69 Catherine M. Butland, 'No. 1 Mobile Military Hospital's journeyings as it affected the sisters, December 1942, to June 1943', MMM QARANC uncatalogued archive MEF memoirs.

70 K.M.C., 'In step with the QAs. 6'. – Blitz on George Cross Island', *Nursing Times* (16 September 1944): 644.

71 Morgan, 'My own dearest Mums', letter 56 (August 1943), CMF, 1.

72 Newlands, *Civilians into Soldiers*, 117.

73 Christine E. Hallett, *Veiled Warriors: Allied Nurses of the First World War* (Oxford, Oxford University Press, 2014), 93–4. The Second World War also experienced typhus epidemics, most notably in Persia and in Naples in the winter of 1943–44. See Jane Brooks 'Nursing typhus victims in the Second World War, 1942–1944', *Journal of Advanced Nursing* 70, 7 (2014): 1510–19; Mark Harrison, *Medicine and Victory: British Military Medicine in the Second World War* (Oxford: Oxford University Press, 2004), 135–7.

74 Joanna Bourke, *The Second World War: A People's History* (Oxford: Oxford University Press, 2001), 126.

75 Harrison, *Medicine and Victory*. See, for example, discussions relating to the work of stretcher-bearers at Monte Cassino, p. 163 and evacuation flights in the monsoon seasons of India and Bengal, p. 226.

76 Kevin Brown, *Fighting Fit: Health, Medicine and War in the Twentieth Century* (Stroud: The History Press, 2008, Kindle edition), loc. 5162; Harrison, *Medicine and Victory*, see especially, for winter conditions in Norway, pp. 38–40, and for tropical campaigns, pp. 95–7.

77 Toman, *Sister Soldiers of the Great War*, 83; Hallett, *Containing Trauma*, 132, 133; Harris, *More than Bombs and Bandages*, loc. 1334.

78 Harris, *More than Bombs and Bandages*, loc. 1326.

79 Mark Harrison, *The Medical War: British Military Medicine in the First World War* (Oxford: Oxford University Press, 2010), 81; Hallett, *Containing Trauma*, 88–9. Trench foot did remain a problem amongst Allied POWs working on the Burma railway. Harrison, *Medicine and Victory*, 78.

80 Wilson, 'We also served, 1940', 29.

81 Bartlett, *Nurse in War*, 108.

82 Nicola Tyrer, *Sisters in Arms: British Army Nurses Tell their Story* (London: Phoenix, 2008), 155.

83 Hutchinson, 'My war and welcome to it', 62.

84 Mary Travis, Territorial Army Nursing Service (TANS), 'General hospital in the desert: Middle East Forces', MMM QARANC/PE/1/320/ WW2.

85 Morgan, 'Still with the lamp', letter 68 (December 1943), 1. CMF, Italy.

86 Anonymous Sister, 'The Anzio beachhead', MMM QARANC uncatalogued archive, CMF file.

87 Sister TANS, 'My experiences in a CCS in the Middle East', MMM QARANC uncatalogued archive, MEF memoirs. Despite the probable dangers of fire, it seems that oil heaters were a common form of heating in tented hospitals throughout the war zones. Sister Winifred Margaret Mountford's (later Winstanley) unpublished memoir also mentions their use in early

1940 when she was part of the British Expeditionary Force in Brittany. I am indebted to Liz Williams for reminiscences of her mother, Winifred Mountford (Monty), who served with the QAs in the UK, northern France and Egypt during the Second World War. E.M. Leeming's (later Wallis) memoir of her war service in Jerusalem also carries a description of oil burners in tented hospitals. E.M. Leeming, 'My war years, 1939–1945', 4, Wellcome Library, London, PP/LEE.

88 Leeming, 'My war years', 3.

89 Underhill, 'To the Matron-in-Chief, Q.A.I.M.N.S.'.

90 Anonymous Sister, 'Middle East and the hospital at Tobruk, December 1939–October 1942', 1, MMM QARANC uncatalogued archive.

91 Low, 'Sudan: 32 General Hospital in the Middle East 1939–1942'.

92 Ana Carden-Coyne, *The Politics of Wounds: Military Patients and Medical Power in the First World War* (Oxford: Oxford University Press, 2014), 198.

93 Bowden, *Grey Touched with Scarlet*, 116.

94 Salter, 'Long ago and far away', 134–5.

95 Harris, *More than Bombs and Bandages*, loc. 1385; Hallett, *Containing Trauma*, 149.

96 L.K. Allen, 'A nursing sister's desert experience with the 8th Army (Africa)', MMM QARANC uncatalogued archive

97 Penny Starns, *Nurses at War: Women on the Frontline, 1939–45* (Stroud: Sutton Publishing, 2000), 46. Although it is acknowledged that many patients and nurses find maggot therapy repugnant, it is one method used in current wound care to clear wounds of 'slough' and promote healing. It is not clear how many ordinary nurses understood its therapeutic benefits in the Second World War. Mortimer cites Barbara Greenwood, a student nurse at the Middlesex Hospital in London, finding a maggoty wound and reporting her horror to the ward sister. The sister was aware of their value and wanted the maggots left. Mortimer, *Sisters*, 88–9. David Justham's analysis of the use of maggots in the Second World War to clean wounds was that they were accidental, considered 'repulsive', but accepted as highly beneficial. David Justham, '"Those maggots – they did a wonderful job": The nurses' role in wound management in civilian hospitals during the Second World War', in Jane Brooks and Christine E. Hallett (eds), *One Hundred Years of Nursing Wartime Practices, 1854–1953* (Manchester: Manchester University Press, 2015), 200.

98 Harrison, *Medicine and Victory*, 86; Hallett, *Containing Trauma*, 132.

99 Morgan, 'Still with the lamp', My own dearest Mums' letter 55 (July1943), 2, MEF.

100 62 Field Hygiene Section, CMF issued in connection with 56 Area Health Week, *Your Other Enemies* (13–19 May 1945), Wellcome Library; Eric Taylor, *Women Who Went to War, 1938–46* (London: Robert Hale, 1988),

128. Taylor acknowledges Marjorie Bennett as one the women who provided either written or recorded information for his book. Information regarding the location of these accounts is not provided. However, he does inform the reader that Sister Bennett's first active service was as part of the British Expeditionary Force to France in January 1940, after which she spent two years in the desert.

101 Anonymous Sister, 'Adventures of a Nursing Officer, 1939–1945 and sidelights of nursing of some tropical diseases, also battle wounds', 12, MMM QARANC uncatalogued archive, MEF memoirs.

102 H.S. Gillespie, 'Some experiences in hospitals in the Middle East, 1939–1942', MMM QARANC uncatalogued archive, MEF memoirs.

103 Sister TANS, 'My experiences in a CCS in the Middle East.

104 Low, 'Sudan, Thirty-two General Hospital in the Middle East, 1939–1942'.

105 Jones, 'Dear mother and father' (1 February 1940), *A Time To Remember*, 21.

106 Nicola Tyrer maintains that the Italians, having considerable experience of desert conditions, were able to prevent such calamities through the use of long poles dug into the sand and external sandbags. The British used pegs and ropes, of little use when the Khamseen wind blew at 50 miles per hour across the desert. Tyrer, *Sisters in Arms*, 153.

107 Newlands, *Civilians into Soldiers*, 65.

108 Bond, *Wartime Experiences from the Midnight Sun*, 23; Collins, 'My dearest Mummy and Daddy' (7 January 1941), 1. See also Brenda McBryde, *A Nurse's War* (Saffron Walden: Cakebread Publications, 1993), 67.

109 Joyce C. Hilder, 'All in the day's work IV. – Darkest Africa!', *Nursing Times* 38, 19 (7 February 1942): 93.

110 There is some discrepancy over this procedure. McBryde maintained that all instruments were 'greased to prevent rust, wrapped in oiled paper, sewn in sacking and packed in crates which were then stencilled with an identifying number'. McBryde, *A Nurse's War*, 67. According to the oral history of Joan Carr, who was also with the QAs in Northern Europe in 1944, the instruments they brought for surgery were not the type that would rust, though she makes no comment about the meticulous packing for quick identification. Joan Carr, oral history interview by Jane Brooks, at her home in the North West, 22 November 2013. Mrs Carr's memory about the events of the Second Front was not excellent, so it is difficult to know if her memory on this matter was accurate or not.

111 After the retreat and virtual surrender of the Italians in February 1941, the Italian Army were reinforced by a German Army Division, under the command of Field Marshal Erwin Rommel. This division would later become the famous Afrika Korps. According to Mark Harrison, the British did not expect a counter-attack from the Germans, leaving themselves tactically weakened. By July 1941, the German advancing force had trapped the British 8th Army at Tobruk in Libya, General Wavell and his reinforce-

ments were defeated and forced to retreat back to Egypt. In late 1941, under General Auchinleck, the British 8th Army in North Africa managed to push Rommel back nearly 400 miles. Despite this partial victory for the British, Rommel's tactics enabled him to regroup and by June 1942 he had recaptured Tobruk. However, after 300 miles of advance into El Alamein in Egypt, Rommel ran out of supplies and no reinforcements came. He could not advance without food, fuel and ammunition, but Hitler had ordered him not to retreat. The British 8th Army, now under the leadership of General Montgomery, attacked El Alamein on 23 October 1942; the battle that ensued lasted ten days. See Harrison, *Medicine and Victory*; James Lucas, *War in the Desert: the Eighth Army at El Alamein* (London: Arms and Armour Press, 1982); Martin Gilbert, *The Second World War: A Complete History* (London: Phoenix, 2009); Richard J. Evans, *The Third Reich at War* (London: Penguin, 2009).

112 Anonymous, '10th C.C.S. at El Alemein [*sic*]', MMM QARANC uncatalogued archive, MEF memoirs

113 Anonymous Sister, 'Adventures of a nursing officer, 1939–1945', 13.

114 Betty Evans, oral history interview by Jane Brooks via telephone, 10 January 2014, UKCHN Archive, University of Manchester .

115 Anonymous Sister, 'Middle East and the hospital at Tobruk'.

116 Mountford, 'Unpublished memoir', 7–9.

117 Ffolliott, 'Account of work and experience in West Africa, May 1941–June 1943'.

118 Allen, 'A nursing sister's desert experience with the 8th Army'.

119 Underhill, 'To the Matron-in-Chief, Q.A.I.M.N.S.'

120 Butland, 'Army sisters in battledress', 64.

121 K.M.C., 'In step with the QAs. 6', 643.

122 Sister TANS, 'My experiences in a CCS in the Middle East'.

123 Ffolliott, 'Account of work and experience in West Africa'.

124 Moody, 'With a pen and brush – a Q.A. reports. 4. – Night duty – with a difference', *Nursing Times* 40, 49 (2 December 1944): 829.

125 Jones, 'My dear mother and father' (25 August 1941), *A Time to Remember*, 125.

126 Low, 'Sudan, Thirty-two General Hospital in the Middle East, 1939–1942'.

127 Betty C. Parkin, *Desert Nurse* (London: Robert Hale, 1990), 101.

128 F.A.E. Crew, *The Army Medical Services: Volume II: Campaigns: Hong Kong, Malaya, Iceland and the Faroes, Libya, 1942–1943, North West Africa* (London: HMSO, 1957), 255.

129 Toman, *An Officer and a Lady*, 109.

130 Allen, *A Nursing Sister's Desert Experience with the 8th Army*.

131 Hilder, 'All in the day's work IV. – Darkest Africa!', 93.

132 Hilder, 'All in the day's work IV. – Darkest Africa!', 93.

133 Newlands, *Civilians into Soldiers*, 162.

134 Crew, *The Army Medical Services: Volume II*, 261.
135 Harrison, *Medicine and Victory*, 109.
136 Santanu Das, *Touch and Intimacy in First World War Literature* (Cambridge: Cambridge University Press, 2005), especially ch. 6, 204–28.
137 Carden-Coyne, *The Politics of Wounds*, see especially ch. 2: 'Surgical wars', 88–139.
138 Harrison, *Medicine and Victory*.
139 Hallett, *Containing Trauma*, 92–101; Toman, *An Officer and a Lady*, especially 124–30; Jan Thore Lockertsen, Ashild Fause, Christine E. Hallett and Jane Brooks, 'The Norwegian Mobile Army Surgical Hospital: Nursing at the front', in Jane Brooks and Christine E. Hallett (eds), *One Hundred Years of Nursing Wartime Practices, 1854–1953* (Manchester: Manchester University Press, 2015); Toman, *Sister Soldiers of the Great War*.
140 Evelyn Pearce, *A General Textbook of Nursing: A Comprehensive Guide to the Final State Examinations* (London: Faber and Faber, 1937), 643.
141 Mogg, 'My work and experiences in the Middle-East. No. 64 General Hospital, Alexandria', MMM QARANC uncatalogued archive. Excerpts of this correspondence to Dame Katherine Jones later appeared in Ada Harrison, *Grey and Scarlet: letters from the war areas by Army Sisters on active service* (London: Hodder and Stoughton, 1943), 128–9.
142 E.L. L'Estrainge, 'Work and experiences in the Middle-East, 1941–1942', MMM QARANC uncatalogued archive, MEF memoirs.
143 Amy Selina (Pam) Dunnett, oral history interview by Lyn E. Smith 25 March 1999, IWM Sound Archive 18784.
144 Lynn Abrams, *Oral History Theory* (London: Routledge, 2010), 83.
145 Dyer, 'When life was grey and scarlet', 51.
146 Dyer, 'When life was grey and scarlet', 70.
147 L'Estrainge, 'Work and experiences in the Middle-East, 1941–1942'.
148 Butland, 'Army sisters in battledress', 11–12.
149 Das, *Touch and Intimacy*, 188.
150 Jeremy A. Crang, '"Come into the Army Maud": Women, military conscription, and the Markham Inquiry', *Defence Studies* 8, 3 (2008): 390.

3

Nursing presence

> Somehow it's more than just good nursing that's required of us, it's endless donkey work and then it's endless interest in the boys and encouragement and jokes, and endless sense of humour, and then there's the job of amusing them when they are getting better and then there's the inevitable letters afterwards![1]

Military success in war was contingent on men sustaining a determination to fight. Persuading men to continue fighting or returning them to combat after illness or injury depended on maintaining their morale. On active service overseas in the Second World War, the use of female nurses in upholding this resolve was integral to the war effort.[2] Military commanders, particularly General Montgomery,[3] appreciated and heralded the placement of female nurses in hospitals in forward areas as a means of 'lifting the lonely soldier's morale'.[4] Military authorities were aware of female nurses as a powerful tool and used their presence as women, especially women from the same nation as the soldiers, as a weapon to encourage the continued participation of men in battle. Nursing sisters' testimonies acknowledge the importance that they, the nurses themselves and their patients, placed on their presence as women, and specifically as 'white women' in the hostile environment of front-line duty. Yet this understanding is on occasion tempered by an acknowledgement that some men saw them as a composite of 'woman', rather than being interested in them 'as an individual'.[5]

War is a gender-destabilising event and, as active participants in it, nurses were caught between wanting to be part of the war effort and to be seen as professional women, and having these aspects of themselves subsumed into that of 'being female'.[6] This led to the precarious image in which nurses' chief contribution to the war effort could be seen in terms of their gender.[7] Nursing sisters in the Second World War were aware of their gendered position as morale boosters, but they did not always see this as a denigration of their professional and clinical skills. They openly used themselves therapeutically within their clinical routines and understood the essential nature of their presence 'when technology reached its limits'.[8]

As British women, nursing sisters acted as constant reminders of wives, daughters and mothers at home, thus ostensibly emulating the traditional family structure supported by politicians and social commentators.[9] This image of domesticity was complicated by the reality that nursing sisters were young women in front-line duties with minimal moral supervision. In order for nurses to be posted into the highly masculine spaces of war, collusion in which both they and their male colleagues exaggerated their femininity was needed,[10] but paradoxically, it was their womanhood that gave rise to anxieties. The presence of women in the masculine world of battle with intimate knowledge of the naked male body intensified fears of moral laxity.[11] Long-standing attitudes towards men's susceptibility to women's sexuality were difficult to erode.[12]

In order to avoid accusations of improper behaviour, the nursing profession had demanded a professional, that is, 'impersonal', relationship with patients.[13] The development of a more human response to the soldiers' sufferings to promote recovery contravened this policy. This chapter examines the nurses' 'use of self' to recover their combatant patients whilst negotiating the realm between the non-sexualised nurse–patient relationship and their presence as women who bolstered men's resolve to fight.[14] The chapter begins with a discussion of the value of the presence of women in hospital wards on active service overseas. It considers the occasional antipathy of military authorities and male colleagues to their location in war zones. However, it is argued that through the provision of expert clinical care, domestic acumen and the use of their 'female selves', nurses were able to salvage men in readiness to return to battle. Nursing sisters thus created a space for themselves in front-line duties. The chapter demonstrates that the use of humour to support healing helped to dispel anxieties about impropriety in the encounter between young single women and vulnerable male soldiers and to further support nurses' presence in the masculine world of war.

The chapter then examines the morale-boosting presence of nurses outside the hospital ward as they became dance partners, dinner guests and potential wives for healthy male members of the allied military. However, inherent in this social 'availability' in a war zone were contraventions of gender, class and racial beliefs of the correct space for white women. Thus, as with their predecessors in the colonial nursing service,[15] the chapter explores their position as single white women in far-flung places. This position situated nurses on active service overseas in a liminal place between the respectable European colonial wife and the 'biohazardous' local women.[16] The chapter acknowledges these difficulties, but also demonstrates how the nurses attempted to use these attributes to their advantage and for those in their care. The final section examines the ramifications of these social relationships on their interactions with their medical officer colleagues. It argues that war required doctors to rethink their understanding of the worth of the nursing staff.

Engaging in caring relationships with very ill patients is highly stressful for nurses.[17] Writing about wars at either end of the twentieth century, Charlotte Dale and Kara Dixon Vuic suggest that sometimes nurses were concerned that acting as female companions potentially denigrated their worth as professional women.[18] The testimonies of nurses for this book suggest that attending parties and social events was a welcome distraction to the arduous work of war nursing and that they enjoyed freedoms that had not been allowed in Britain.[19] Although some nurses came from the same social class as their male officer colleagues, as more and more nurses were needed and thus integrated into the military, the class basis of the army nurse necessarily expanded. In *Creating Rosie the Riveter*, gender historian Maureen Honey argues that women's magazines in the USA, cognisant of the limited opportunities for women's professional success, sold upward mobility through the marriage market, usually by marrying the boss.[20] Many nursing sisters were not blind to the social contract that they could make on active service overseas, but it was not without its difficulties. As an Irish Catholic, Sister Mary Morris was honest in her reflections on her impending marriage to Malcolm, with his Church of England and middle-class roots. She wrote of the difference in their social and religious backgrounds, 'Will we be able to overcome the problems of our different cultures?'[21] The contract, however, generally benefitted both parties; male officer gained a useful wife and the nurse gained social mobility, 'or at least alleviation from the monotony of military life'.[22] Nurses used this social aspect of their presence not only to negotiate their relationships with male officers in general, but to renegotiate their relationships with male medical officers in particular.

Nursing presence on hospital wards

Penny Summerfield identifies the complexities in the delineation of 'woman' as a feminine ideal, where 'femininity' itself is 'unstable and problematic'.[23] The position of women in war heightens the multiple discourses of femininity, especially for nurses on active service overseas. Nurses were involved in a complex interplay in which they were the epitome of the feminised worker, located in the least female of spaces and where the exigencies of war placed numerous demands on them as professional workers, soldiers, mothers, lovers and daughters.[24] It was never entirely possible to harmonise these various demands that had been placed on them by military commanders and society in general.[25] Even in a highly mobile war the expectation was that nurses, as women, would be kept away from combat, yet as nurses their skills were needed close to the front line. Ultimately, whatever the political rhetoric about the safety of women in war, trained nurses' skills were essential in combat zones to salvage soldiers.[26] Despite this, they still needed to broker careful gender negotiations on active service overseas to ensure their place at the front.

In July 1943 Sister Agnes Morgan wrote to her mother that although she felt 'so altogether helpless in the face of this tide of human suffering',[27] she begged her not to ask her to return home: 'I wish that you could just see "my boys" for one minute. You wouldn't want me to leave them for 1 minute or 1 hour, let alone altogether! How would I know that anybody else had remembered to feed my poor "broken backs", how would I know that the poor crippled legs had their pillows just "fixed".'[28] In the autumn of 1944 Sister Penny Salter and her colleagues were posted to a rapidly created field hospital on the Burma Road to care for soldiers in the middle of an outbreak of scrub typhus.[29] When they were within the vicinity of the hospital, but at this point quite lost, they were met by members of the Military Police, who clearly did not believe their story:

> 'Then, who do you think we are?' I [Salter] repeated. 'You could be anyone' he mumbled under his breath, 'and as for a hospital in this area – impossible'. 'Very well, have it your own way,' I replied, 'But first of all explain why you say it is impossible'. 'For one thing', he said, 'It is inconceivable to have a hospital in this area with Q/As. Secondly, we would have been the first to have been informed had there been a front line hospital set up – 'But why no Q/As', I insisted – he paused, and then grunting said, 'It is far too forward and dangerous for any Q/As to be working here at the moment.' 'But surely someone has to nurse the troops, and who better than us?'[30]

When they eventually arrived on the hospital wards they found, 'just boys, nothing but skin and bone, physically and mentally sick'.[31] Salter continued that on seeing the nurses enter the ward with the colonel, the soldier-patients:

> Whisper in hushed and muted tones, 'White sisters, Q/As from home. Are they real?'. Yes we were real, very real, so real that even we were moved to tears. Three days later there was laughter and wise cracks heard in the ward; the moral [*sic*] of the men on the mend, and all because of a handful of nursing sisters from home flitted around the wards. Having finished our round with the colonel we went off and met the doctors who were far too few and grossly overworked. Not being au fait with scrub typhus we were eager to obtain some knowledge of this disease.[32]

The recovery work of nurses on active service overseas in CCSs, field units – such as the one to which Salter was posted – and base hospitals was a combination of clinical skill and their use of self, most particularly the use of their female self. In the mid-twentieth century, nurses did not see their position as women as a devaluation of their worth, but rather as part of their importance in a war zone. Nurses were keen to demonstrate their skills as professional women and officers and to raise their status in the armed forces; critical to these ambitions was their placement on the front line. They were also aware that in order to have access to this privileged male domain, they needed to accept that their body and presence would be used as part of any acknowledged litany of their skills.[33] When the nurses

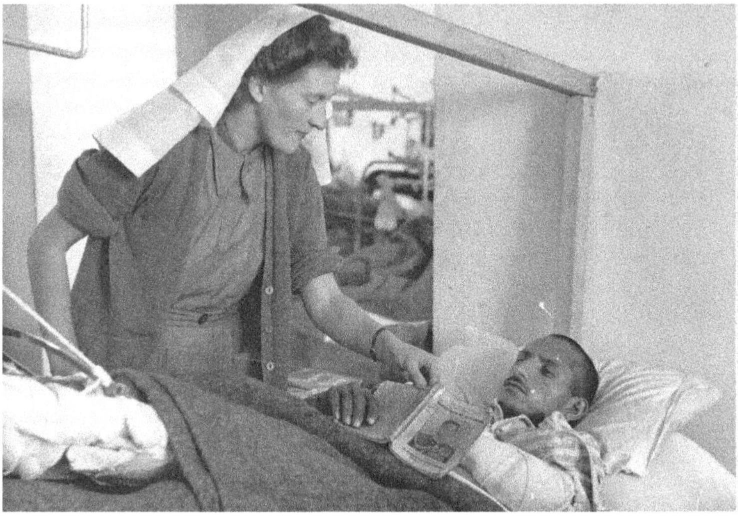

6 An older nurse during a quiet moment with a patient.

wrote of the helplessness of their combatant patients and that they are just 'boys', the reader is drawn both to the youth of the soldier, their need for a mother figure and the potential of impropriety that the proximity of young men to young single women raises. In using themselves as part of the recovery process, the complexity of the position of female nurses in war zones was intensified.

'War is a man's business'

The belief that nurses should be in forward areas was 'proven' in the First World War. Authorities were not blind to the improvement in the troops' morale because of the presence of nurses, partly through nurses simply 'being there'[34] and partly through the soon recognised 'indispensability'[35] of their skills in 'supportive care'.[36] By the Second World War, nurses were considered essential participants in war. According to Sister Brenda McBryde, General Montgomery was more than aware of the advantages to the men in having female nursing sisters caring for them, even if that meant having women in forward areas.[37] As one nurse maintained, the morale of the troops was raised 'the moment they saw the nursing sisters'.[38] However, there were many male members of the military who were not convinced that female nurses should be in forward areas. Lucy Noakes argues that women in combat positions in war are of particular concern, as 'combat is "naturally" a male occupation' and the 'presence of women threatens the masculine cohesion and efficiency of combat units'.[39] She refers to John Laffin's ideology that 'war is a man's business'.[40] Nurses may not have been in combat positions, but by posting them en masse to forward areas the authorities placed them in danger.

Both PMRAFNS Sister Iris Bower and QA Sister Mary Morris recalled the antipathy towards the nursing sisters going to Normandy in June 1944. However, in both cases the irritation that women had the 'temerity [to enter] … this "man's" world'[41] was tempered with more prosaic issues than the presence of female nurses in a war zone. In Bower's case the issue seemed to be one of lack of lavatories for her and her colleague Mollie.[42] In some instances the antipathy carried with it more serious undertones of what it was acceptable for women to do in war and when they could do it.[43] Not all medical officers were unequivocal in their praise of nurses.[44] Dr George Feggetter, RAMC, wrote in his diary that following his arrival in Algiers in October 1942 as part of Operation Torch, 'There is no doubt that the presence of female nurses on the day of the landing and for three or four weeks afterwards would have been a handicap in the immediate treatment and care of the wounded.'[45] Occasionally the hostility towards the nurses created a situation where instead of respecting the accepted trope that women should be protected, male military colleagues left the nurses to fend for themselves. When Germany invaded Greece in April 1941, the hospital in which Sister Jessie Wilson was working was forced to evacuate: 'At 4.0pm, one of the Sisters came over and said that the Colonel and Registrar had gone with the men … We could not believe it, – a handful of M.O.s and orderlies and 40 women left alone, – and I think for the first time we felt a bit scared.'[46]

The nursing sisters of the Second World War were nevertheless determined to be part of the war effort. They knew that they had the requisite clinical skills that they believed would be invaluable in forward areas supporting the recovery of troops. Whilst it was their gender that could stymie their access to front-line duties, they soon realised that it was also their ticket. Sister Evelyn Cottrell recalled a colonel telling them that the battle for Monte Cassino would be a brutal one and they did not have to go, 'but of course everybody went, you couldn't imagine us saying we wouldn't go'.[47] In the absence of sufficient medical officers, nurses were needed to give blood transfusions, remove shrapnel from wounds and perform minor surgery.[48] Sister Elsie Driver was with a contingent of nurses posted from North Africa to Italy following the Salerno landings in September 1943. She and her colleagues expressed indignation when they were initially prevented from going ashore because the officers were unhappy about women entering a war zone.[49] According to Jean Bowden, the matron spoke for all of them when she maintained that 'we all feel that it would be wasteful to have brought us this far and not use us'. The next morning they landed on Italian soil and within one hour were setting up a hospital in a ruined school building and admitting convoys of men: 'The men on stretchers, desperately wounded though they were, heaved themselves up on an elbow to see the truth of the shout that went up: "Women! English sisters – here already".'[50] In such cases the benefit to the sick and injured troops of British nursing sisters simply being there seemed to be greater than any treatment

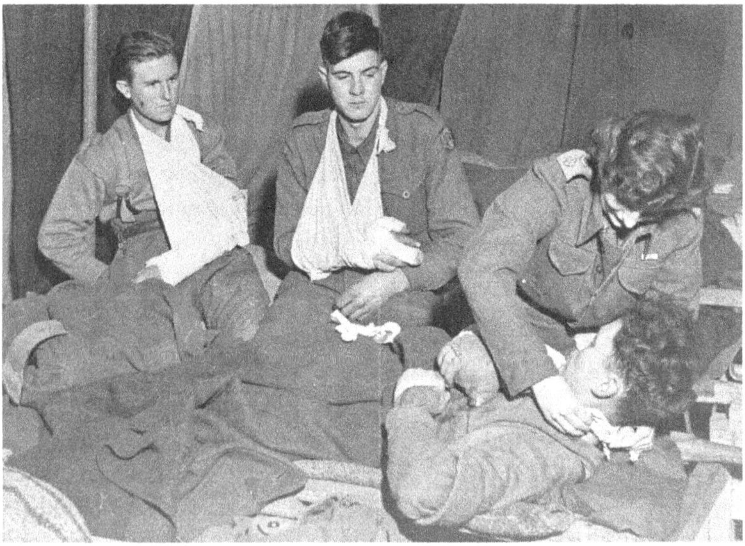

7 Field Hospital, Italy. A nurse demonstrates her clinical nursing skills. Note the compassion with which they were performed and the avid interest of the watching soldiers.

that could be offered. Butland admitted in her unpublished memoir that often men did not really need treatment at all, they just needed to talk to a woman.[51]

The nurses thus parlayed both their clinical skills and their gendered identity to pursue war careers on the front line, in spaces that had hitherto been essentially male places. Their presence in war zones, if veiled from the public at home, developed into an accepted and acceptable nursing space. Butland and Wilson even believed that despite front-line postings potentially usurping the work of orderlies, even they began to view having female nurses as beneficial to patient care.[52]

'The patients were amazed to see us'

Margarete Sandelowski argues that, into the twentieth century, the 'body of the nurse was still the most important tool in her growing armamentarium',[53] thus her very physical being was a central aspect to her nursing work. In August 1944 the *Nursing Times* reprinted a letter from one officer patient to his wife: 'I have been deeply moved at the tenderness of a man [RAMC orderly] to a man, but the QAs bring more than tenderness. No more strategically intelligent order was ever given than to send the QAs to the beachhead. The morale of a desperate venture was injected with a new vitality.'[54] The nurses' presence both calmed the men who were too ill to fight and also created an environment in which men's morale was raised. In a letter to her mother, Sister Pat Moody stated that 'one feels that one is really doing something for the poor devils. I don't think they would be nearly so comfortable if we weren't here, which is some consolation.'[55] Sister Francie E. Brown recalled one particularly nervous patient who 'depended on me absolutely'.[56] Morris marvelled at the delight of the family atmosphere on her ward,[57] and several sisters recalled the joy and 'wonder' the troops expressed when they were cared for by female sisters in forward hospitals.[58] Sister L.K. Allen wrote to Dame Katharine Jones of the build-up to the battle of El Alamein, which began on 23 October 1942:

> Field Marshall Montgomery was all set with plans laid out, not only for the men to fight but for the sick and wounded to be cared for just behind the lines, so for the first time in history Army Sisters were allowed to go deep into the Desert following close behind the advancing 8th Army … when

the men first encountered the Sisters in the Desert it was so amusing to see their goggle eyed, open mouthed expressions, which suddenly changed into a broad grin and then – A loud cheer.[59]

One nursing sister on the Anzio beachhead wrote of the responsiveness of the troops, 'possibly more so because one and all they seemed amazed to find sisters so far forward. I remember going into a tent one day, dressed as usual in battledress and tin hat, trouser-legs tucked into gum boots. As I was talking to a patient, I heard a husky whisper behind – "Gorblimey! It's a nurse".'[60] When Butland made her morning round on her first day at a hospital near Benghazi:

The patients were amazed to see us … We heard comments to the effect that all would now be well. That the Army couldn't retreat now it had its Sisters up in the forward areas … The next morning when I did a hospital round the patients all said how much better they felt from only just seeing Sisters about the hospital.[61]

It is highly probable that nurses' testimonies would identify the criticality of their presence as part of the war effort, given the prospects for their professional status that could come from such encounters. However, it was not only the nurses themselves who wrote of the importance of their placement in hospital wards across the globe. An American medical officer who had been a patient with the 99th General Hospital, British North African campaign wrote that 'they [British nurses] are kind, efficient, and goodhearted. Gosh, nothing is too much trouble.'[62] In his memoir, *My Moving Tent: Diary of a Desert Rat*, A.A. Nicol described the nursing sisters moving 'quietly between beds where lay the helpless wounded'. He continued by stating that 'it was particularly soothing to see their dim figures moving about in the shadows while the building shook and shuddered to the fall of bombs and the rage of guns outside'.[63]

Although physicians on active service overseas were aware that the male orderlies were in many ways willing and able nurses, there was a belief that 'the patients seem to do better practically and psychologically when sisters were there'.[64] The chief commendation of Dr Feggetter went to the work of orderlies, whom he described as doing the work 'to the best of their ability with great solicitude'. However, even he admitted that when the sisters arrived, although he did not think that 'a single man had been adversely affected in any way by the absence of the QAs … the art of nursing was not so evident'.[65] Arguably it was this art, or artistry of the female nurses' work and their presence at the bedside that acted as a supporter of healing and recovery.[66] Their expert nursing and compassionate care also brought gratitude from mothers, fathers and wives at home, engendering a confidence in the management of the sick and injured on the home front as well as the front line.[67] Such was the importance of the location of nurses in war zones that it stayed with patients even until after the war.

'Fun, and honest interest'

In September 1945, David Emery wrote to Butland, reminiscing about his time in a desert hospital: 'An injured man is often a very weak creature. He feels very alone and quite sorry for himself … You folks, however, with your scolding, fun, and honest interest, give the patient the feeling somebody cares about him, is expecting him to get well.'[68] Notwithstanding Feggetter's commendation that nursing sisters demonstrated art in their work, he also maintained that the nurses' presence created stricter discipline and a less easy atmosphere.[69] The majority of the nurses' personal testimonies, whilst acknowledging that their matrons may have expected more formal care practices, do not suggest a strict discipline on their wards; in fact the opposite seems to have been the case. Their writings and those of their patients, like David Emery's above, point to the use of humour both as a method of recovery work and to dispel the spectre of impropriety. The use of humour and fun took a number of different guises. Sometimes the nurses themselves promoted the fun, sometimes they accepted that it was they who were the object of fun and sometimes they simply allowed it to happen. In some instances relationships with their patients should have been built before humour could be used to good effect. Where relationships were presumed, the comedy could backfire. Sister P.M. Dyer wrote in her diary of a practical joke they played on one 'handsome blond young officer' patient on whom, whilst he was still unconscious from the anaesthetic, they 'set to with all the aids required for female vanity, gave his face a "New Look"'. When he awoke he was apparently not at all amused, although Dyer admits that they became firm friends.[70] Thus, even when the humour was not initially welcome, it could act as a part of the method that creates a valuable nurse–patient relationship and therefore one that could support recovery and enable nurses to conduct emotionally challenging work.[71]

In her oral history interview Marion Cash maintains that in hospitals on the home front the nurses enjoyed the company of their combatant patients, but were not allowed to be frivolous with them and had to always call them by their surnames.[72] It seems as if even on the home front, by the end of the war this had changed in some hospitals.[73] As early as the First World War, the use of humour, and especially laughter, was openly supported. Staff and patients saw its importance for crossing class and gender boundaries and therefore dissipating the potential difficulties present in a military hospital.[74] There was a general acceptance that it created cohesiveness between patients and nurses, alleviating stressful situations,[75] enhancing well-being, reducing pain and assisting patients to manage the fears of illness.[76]

One nursing sister at the Anzio beachhead wrote that, despite the pain, 'there were lots of smiling faces and jokes passed'.[77] Morgan wrote of the 'great jokes' she had with her patients, 'and plenty of cheerful conversation'.[78] Morris in her multinational ward in Normandy in July 1944 wrote that she 'could never run this ward without the lovely spirit of warm friendliness which exists between all of us. They like to tease me and I like to encourage their involvement with each other.'[79] Much of this cheerfulness apparently came from 'a game called "Housey Housey"' that they played for hours. 'It is noisy and cheerful and hilariously funny because of the language barriers … It is lovely to see how the players try to involve the [shell] shocked ones like Lt Martin with encouraging remarks of "have a go mate", "pulling rank" is not "on" here.'[80] Fortunately for Morris, her matron, Miss Wade, 'turned a blind eye to the chaos. We do all we can to make the boys happy as possible.'[81] Sister Mary Bond recalled one improvised concert for the sick troops during which their matron and commanding officer (CO) joined in with the singing and actions to the songs.[82]

Not all matrons were so amenable to such levels of fraternisation. Bower's matron was not at all amused when she heard the troops calling out to Bower using her nickname 'Fluffy'.[83] There was a clear rationale for a non-fraternisation policy. Ana Carden-Coyne notes the extreme difficulties in the First World War when doctors became too close to troops and then were required to make triage decisions.[84] Nevertheless, it seems that the nurses and their medical colleagues, including those in senior positions, were aware of the value of fun and supported their soldier-patients' amusing themselves and laughing as much as possible.[85] Roberta Love Tayloe, an America nurse with the 9th Evacuation Hospital (field hospital) described her tent of 'lively officers' who decided to write a film: 'I was delighted with the movie project. It kept them amused. The story went, "this beautiful nurse was kidnapped by a German. He just grabbed her up screaming, tucked her under his arm and sped away in his tank".'[86] Sister Betty Parkin's memoirs recall her 'ballet' performance in a hospital in Egypt on Boxing Day 1940, an event which she clearly believed was excellent respite for the patients:

> 'The sisters will dance for us' … in response to this announcement, shouts and whistles broke out … Regardless that the opening bars of 'The Skaters' Waltz' had yet to be played, the first of my *corps de ballet* bounded onto the stage – the rest followed, their steps badly mixed as they tried to pick up the music. The 'counter' coming last, gasped between her '1, 2, 3': 'You're all going the wrong way. You're doing the wrong steps'. The audience roared with laughter … After entering the first ward that evening I decided to leave the rest to the orderlies until all were settled. Men had leapt forward to strike ballet poses, and a trio perched precariously on a bed were using a mosquito net as a stage curtain. Next morning one of the wards presented me with a silver paper crown and wand.[87]

One of Morgan's letters in August 1944 exemplifies the importance placed on the soldier-patients' ability to maintain good cheer. Despite being 'still dazed from the Battle, they are cheerful and joky [*sic*] and full of marvellous spirit. I think the thing I like the best is the way they help each other.'[88] Wilson recalled the men on her ward in Egypt teasing her mercilessly: 'I walked down the ward to the sterilising room, when the men started to whistle in time to my footsteps – they knew this infuriated me. When I changed my step, they changed their tempo, until the whole ward was whistling, and I was almost dancing with rage. Soon the men were rocking with laughter, and so was I.'[89] The farewell letter of a Tank Major to Sister Kitty O'Connor sums up the benefits of humour. He had only made it, he said, because of the 'marvellous musical-comedy atmosphere of the ward'.[90] Even when the fun was inappropriate, the nurses wrote of the jokes with amusement. Sister Anne Radloff's soldier-patients took great amusement in teaching the Flemish 'peasant girls' who were acting as nursing assistants vulgar English words, until the hospital authorities put an end to the behaviour.[91] Given the highly stressful and difficult situation of a war zone it is not surprising that the nurses used humour not only to cope with the present, but also to encourage hope in the future. Humour was used as a tool to maintain their patients' sense of personhood.[92] As civilians became soldiers they were subsumed into the machinery of war.[93] The preservation of being human could support their belief in how life would be after war and enable those involved in war to carry on. Nurses were therefore important to maintaining humanity not only in the hospital wards, but also in the wider war community.

Nurses' presence outside the hospital wards

The use of nurses as 'political tools' – emblems for a just war – may not have been a conscious decision. However, the authorities realised that whether they were patients in a hospital ward or fit men awaiting battle, even seeing women in a war zone could remind the men of why they were fighting. The placing of nurses in the most hostile environments of the Second World War therefore worked as fuel to enable the soldiers to continue the battle. Even if the nurses did not understand their presence in this way, they were aware of their power as women from the men's home nation, realising that in some circumstances they were the first women whom the men 'had seen for many months'.[94]

'Pardon me … I haven't seen a woman for over ten months'

The vision of the female nurse in all theatres of war raised the spirits of the men, and the nurses used this to their advantage. If the men were thrilled to see them, then the nursing sisters should be in forward areas to maintain morale. In a report for the BBC on 20 June 1944, correspondent Colin Wells described the arrival of British nurses in Normandy: '"There are", he said, "two days in this war which the British Tommy will never forget. The day he landed and the day 'the ladies' landed. And the ladies were the first nursing officers to come to France. The effect of the nurses' arrival on the *morale* of the troops has been superb".'[95] Sister Emily Soper recalled arriving in Normandy that same summer, 'so we came down onto the beach, we walked up the beach and there were lorries waiting for us, and er, so we went up to the lorries and we were going along and there were soldiers standing around and they cheered us, so that was really quite exciting for us, 'cause we were all just young women'.[96] Butland recalled the surprise of the soldiers when meeting nursing sisters so far forward and maintained that it was with a sense of pride that she and her colleagues happily removed their scarves so 'the men would believe we really were women'.[97]

Being women, and therefore active reminders of home and the reasons why the men were fighting, was a significant aspect to managing the well-being of the men with whom the nurses worked.[98] Radloff maintained that 'Monty thought that the men needed "a little feminity [*sic*]"'.[99] Nurses were arguably complicit in the importance placed on their gender, seeing it as a method of promoting the well-being of the troops. They understood that the benefits of their presence in war zones moved beyond the walls of hospital wards.[100] One nursing sister described the troops making a 'great fuss of us and whenever we wished to travel, we had only to walk along the road and the first Military vehicle that came along would be sure to offer a lift'.[101] An acting matron wrote to Dame Katharine Jones recalling, 'he [the soldier] then stepped back and saluted, saying, "Pardon me, but I thought I must have had one over the eight last night; I haven't seen a woman for over ten months" … Several lorries, armoured cars, etc., were slowed down in order that the occupants could satisfy themselves that we were really women.'[102] Sister Vera Jones recalled the 'great stir when we all arrived [in Palestine] from England, or "Blighty" as the boys call it'.[103] A sister arriving in Tobruk with her colleagues recalled how they were 'enthusiastically entertained by the Brigadier and headquarters' staff of the South African Army'.[104] Another wrote of the wonderful treatment they had received from everyone since they had landed in Durban: 'no one seems able to do enough for us here'.[105] When Salter arrived in Madras with her nurse colleagues on their way to Burma, one high-ranking officer was so keen for their company that he ordered a lunch party for them with chilled wine, liqueurs and coffee and, on their exit, 'the whole restaurant of guests rose to their feet and gave us a standing ovation'.[106] In one of her early letters to her mother, Morgan wrote of the 'necessity' of their presence in war zones. Whether the men arrived at the hospital simply for female company, because they needed treatment for injury or illness, or just on their way to a new posting, the nurses, she wrote, were obligated to always 'make ourselves adequate for the task'.[107]

Army nursing sisters were therefore not blind to the difficulties that arose from this role. Many of the testimonies offer the reader a gilded version of life on active service overseas, with parties and fun and often glorious weather. But, occasionally, letters and diaries provide a darker side to the social life of military nurses. Sister Betty Evans felt that the war was both an adventure and a great cause of sadness when men whom the nurses had travelled with arrived at a hospital or CCS in the dreadful state they so often did.[108] Morgan wrote:

> 'Monty' [General Montgomery] says, 'I hope that the sisters will co-operate in helping to entertain the Victorious 8th Army during their short periods of rest'!! And 'they' certainly did their best – ten of us turned up to the first dance, and had one of the most enjoyable times we've ever had in our lives! Not that it was all pure enjoyment, far from it, very often my eyes filled with tears and my heart near to breaking when I think of the tragedy of War. – all these splendid men and boys who two years ago (or three) were the flower of England's manhood, are now hard-bitten, often bitter, weary-eyed men, going patiently on from day to day, from month to month, seeing no end.[109]

The discussions of the devil-may-care attitude of pilots and their need for the company of nurses invoke a particular sense of pathos. Salter wrote of an encounter with the RAF in Karachi and the squadron leader's decision to give a party for the sisters, despite the duty officer forbidding it: '"Who did they think they were these young airmen"… but these men could not have cared less, they had nothing to lose, except maybe their lives shortly when being shot up over the jungles of Burma.'[110] Wilson was posted to a hospital near Piraeus and noted that the RAF was stationed close by: 'They were just young boys, eager and enthusiastic. One by one they went on flights and never returned.'[111] Although they were near to the fighting in Creully, on 21 June 1944 Morris's matron agreed that the nursing sisters could all go to an RAF dance:

> The boys in blue looked very dashing, particularly 'fighter command' with their long moustaches and top tunic button undone (memories of the Battle of Britain). Such studied nonchalance, very impressive. They had to work hard to impress us actually as there were at least ten of them to each one of us. It is quite exciting to be surrounded by so many men who obviously feel the need for female company. They spoiled us beautifully and we danced and laughed with all of them. Transient fleeting friendships are a part of war. There is never enough time to get to know anybody, and for some there may not be a tomorrow.[112]

Female nurses as 'fair game'

War is alleged to be a highly erotic and exciting time that 'compromise[s] the norms of both femininity and masculinity'.[113] In reality, before the advent of the contraceptive pill, despite the increased freedoms experienced by young single women it was perhaps more a time of romance than sex.[114] In her analysis of the hospital environment in the First World War, Carden-Coyne argues that 'sexual fantasies were part of the ward culture'.[115] Volunteer nurses from middle- and upper-class backgrounds who had been imbued with the ideal of romanticism were perhaps more prone to the draw of the romantic ideal of the injured soldier,[116] as they, the '"weaker sex" dealt with helpless male patients'.[117] Carden-Coyne does not identify any complaints of actual unwanted sexual advances, although this may have been out of embarrassment rather than lack of incidents; nevertheless, military hospitals could be sexually electric places.[118] In *Containing Trauma*, Christine Hallett maintains that the professional nurses were more alert to the 'dangers of "flirtation"' between patients and themselves.[119] By the Second World War, 20 years later, nurses were armed with both registered nurse status and equality of franchise, moves which helped to vindicate their professional position. Sister Nell Jarrett's Second World War diary demonstrated this less guileless and more professional response when she acknowledged the problem of 'sex starvation in the M.E.F. I may be hard but maybe they dwell too much on the situation. At present at any rate I feel no way inclined to do anything to alleviate the situation.'[120]

If girls were generally 'protected' prior to the commencement of the Second World War, the challenges to life caused by bombs and the requirement for young single women to take on roles such as fire watching and anti-aircraft duties altered the attitudes towards risky behaviour.[121] Despite the appreciation of the freedoms this brought young women, the changes in attitudes to sexualised behaviour could promote a more 'dangerous' atmosphere for hospital nurses, rather than sexual equality. Emily Mayhew, Liz Byrski and Julie Anderson demonstrate that whilst nurses increased the range and complexity of their technical nursing work on the home front in Second World War, this did not carry with it an attendant alteration in attitudes and behaviour to the treatment of nurses as women.[122] Byrski examines the position of the nursing staff on the burns ward at East Grinstead Hospital. She maintains that Archibald McIndoe was a misogynist and that there was general acquiescence that female nurses could be sacrificed for the greater good of the men.[123] According to Anderson, it was not only McIndoe who believed this. She argues that the War Office and Winston Churchill himself considered 'the burned pilots behaviour at East Grinstead was to be tolerated and indulged', even if this ignored the sexual harassment of the nurses.[124] The nurses were therefore expected to accept sexual advances and harassment from the doctors and patients alike.

Although few nurses wished to discuss this less savoury aspect of the utility of their female selves as part of the war effort, it is clear that there were members of the military of all ranks who considered them 'fair game'.[125] In her wartime memoir, American nurse LaVonne Telshaw Camp wrote of the 'philandering men in the military and a few impudent officers who felt that the nurses were sent overseas for their own personal comfort and pleasure, and were indignant when these women let them know otherwise'.[126]

Although many nurses' testimonies suggest that they were happy to be considered morale boosters for the troops and many did enjoy the parties, the constant demand to be dance partners for the officers, with or without unwanted sexual advances, could be exhausting.[127] Sister Jane Forrest recollected: 'The officers in the surrounding district tried to keep us lively by entertaining for [*sic*] us. Nearly every Mess gave a Dance and Supper and I have spent some enjoyable evenings in that way.' However, eventually, Forrest admits, they became bored with the endless parties and the one hotel available for supper and stopped going out so much – for which they accrued the name the 'Shaiba snobs'.[128] Jarrett was unequivocal in her views of the demands made by some officers. On 6 September 1942 her diary states that she went out one evening with fellow nursing colleagues as guests of a major and two captains: 'I'd no wish to drink and they thought me sticky. They were so obviously out for all they could get.'[129] Betty Crisp and Margaret Parkes, nurses working on the home front during the war, described difficulties in Britain with both British and US forces' personnel. Crisp recalled an unpleasant situation with some drunken US soldiers in Exeter.[130] Parkes described her vivid memories of a party at an airbase. The soldiers, she said, 'tried to get you up against the wall, they considered you "fair game"'.[131] Parkes argued that although this treatment was meted out to nurses in the UK, troops on active service overseas had only the highest regard for the nursing sisters. She believed that she and her colleagues in Britain were treated like cannon fodder, the sisters on active service overseas as professionals and officers. The distinctions in reality were not so stark, and it is likely that Parkes' and Crisp's memories of the treatment that they experienced were coloured by anxieties about the correct way young women should behave.[132]

Nurses experienced the full range of men's attitudes and behaviour towards them both at home and on active service overseas, from what Telshaw Camp described as 'certain rapacious military men'[133] to the respect and collegiality described by Salter.[134] It is not clear whether Telshaw Camp's comments reflect more on North American servicemen as compared their British counterparts, or whether they simply reflect the differences in men's attitudes to nurses and women more generally. Parkes' shock at the behaviour of servicemen at parties on the airbase for both the RAF and US Air Force made no comment about whether this conduct applied to men from the USA or Britain or both.[135]

Despite these testimonies to less welcome attentions, most nurses on active service overseas appear to have experienced camaraderie with officer colleagues. They appreciated the respite from emotionally charged work that parties with them offered. Thus, whilst some of the personal testimonies do allude to inappropriate sexual expectations both on and off duty, mostly their relationships with male colleagues seem to have been a positive experience. Given the ratio of women to men overseas, and nurses being able to choose between any number of available male officers, a more judicious and less predatory approach from the men was perhaps to be expected. Nurses as officers and, until 1943, often the only single women in far-flung war zones, could pick and choose their partners. Male officers who did not treat the nursing sisters with respect would find themselves without female company, or worse. One doctor, who Sister Catherine Hutchinson felt had touched her inappropriately, was posted elsewhere.[136] But such unsupervised proximity to men in places such as the Far East or Middle Eastern desert, long understood as redolent with romance and potentially unrestrained sexuality, created yet a further layer of complexity for the position of the female nurse.

'The angel in the house'

In one of her letters home from Sierra Leone, Sister Barbara Collins remarked that 'It really is pathetic how eager the batchelors [*sic*] of the Civil Service are for our company & I guess this has gone to the girls' heads a bit!'.[137] The placing of white nurses in the tropics had been a key strategy of colonialism, 'to support the health of white colonists'.[138] The Colonial Nursing Association had been sending its members to Africa, the West Indies and the Indian subcontinent since the later years of the nineteenth century.[139] The desire for the presence of European women in colonised lands as 'the angel in the house', to act as the arbiter of all that was modest, was crucial to the colonial project.[140] They were the 'bearers of racialised heteronormative traditions and feminine respectability'.[141] However, the presence of women in these faraway places was contradictory: 'The colonial nurse, though ostensibly employed to create an ordered hygienic and traditionally "British" treatment environment within the colony, was also a potentially transgressive figure – a single woman travelling to the outposts of empire and encountering unusual challenges and trials due to her situation.'[142] Placing 'British women on the frontiers of the empire', whether as colonial or war nurse, required qualities in them that were frequently 'far from feminine'.[143] Just as their gender was crucial to the colonial project, the criticality of the nurse as woman was retained as they became agents in war. Their womanhood may have been the attribute that raised concerns about their presence, especially anxieties in relation to 'the control of white *women's* sexuality',[144] but it was also the reason for their presence: 'Gender thus functioned as a form of power for women who relied on feminine ideals to justify their place as wartime nurses.'[145]

In far-flung theatres of war, fears that troops would turn to local women for pleasure further promoted calls for the presence of the civilising effect of white women. On overseas duty many men contracted venereal disease (VD) from 'amateur prostitutes' in the cities of North Africa.[146] Figures for the contraction of VD in that area were recorded as being as high as 30 out of every 1,000 soldiers.[147] VDs in some theatres of war were 'almost inexorable', high rates being noted in India in 1943 during the Bengal famine, and in Italy as the allied troops moved up to Rome in 1944.[148] Concerns over the numbers of troops accessing sexual encounters with local women were therefore understandable, especially before the widespread availability of penicillin. The desire to control such high rates of infection, which removed men from duty, was logical. Providing allied soldiers with the vision of the pure white woman, in contrast to the 'unrestrained African female sexuality',[149] would, it was believed, have a civilising effect on men's potential sexual transgressions.[150] Ironically, however, nursing sisters, as officers in the British Army, were not allowed to consort with enlisted men[151] and, although there were occasional romances, enlisted men knew that the nurses were out of bounds.[152] There is evidence that dances were organised between non-commissioned officers and nursing sisters, but relationships outside that highly circumscribed arena were forbidden.[153] Thus, any desires that the military may have had to create 'some wholesome forms of recreation',[154] were made obsolete in practice.

Nursing sisters had a place in far-flung war zones partly to occupy the military and colonial officers and provide, if nothing else, at least an image of pure womanhood to the troops. Yasmin Khan argues that '"Supplying" nurses and Red Cross workers from the USA, Britain, Canada and other white dominions was central to the comforting and healing of men stationed for a long time in an imperial war zone far from home.'[155] But such practices only opened up a realm of inconsistencies for nurses. As young single women who had precocious knowledge of the male body, they were open to criticisms that they were part of the potentially corruptible youth rather than the professional class, whose role it was to curtail and manage sexual profligacy. Such contradictions were essentially bound in the female nurses' use of self. Was her use of self about her as a woman, or as a professional being who healed the wounded and provided expert clinical care and management of the sick? The nurses appear to have understood their place as a combination of woman and clinical expert, but the ambiguities of their position necessitated careful gender and professional brokery. Nevertheless, as Lucy Noakes acknowledges, nursing was considered an acceptable manner in which women could become involved in war.[156] Important for this narrative was the use the female nurses made of the ambiguities of their position. They promoted themselves as 'healthcare professionals and ranking officers, as well as white women', to gain access to ill and injured troops in dangerous places.[157]

In the early years of the twentieth century, the location of nurses in far-flung spaces of the empire 'to carry out the work of healing' was acceptable, so long as it was done 'at a discreet distance' from the war itself. By the Second World War, such geographic demarcations were neither desirable nor possible.[158] The professional nurses of the Second World War had no such notions of ethereal beauty about their work, nor ideas of 'sacrifice',[159] but a belief in the reality of the work they could do and that their position in forward areas was of benefit to the troops. Yet there remained areas in which they could never justify their presence. When Salter was posted to India, she wrote that they worked from eight in the morning till sunset, 'and then handed over to the doctor or ward master on duty as it was taboo for us to be on the wards during the hours of darkness, apart from a quick visit to tend an exceptionally ill patient'.[160] At the end of the war, Radloff was posted to the Indian Medical Services to nurse Indian POWs returned from Japanese camps. Instead of wearing the khaki battle-dress in which she had spent her previous posting, she and her colleagues now 'swanned around in white dresses and shoes. It wasn't done for white women to be seen to be working physically hard.'[161]

Despite the largely racially motivated prohibitions over certain areas of work, the presence of British nurses in war zones was important for both sick and healthy troops, but it was also important for the nurses as professionals. The rapid mobility of the Second World War gave rise to the constant shifting of battle lines. The nature of injury, illness and the importance of the troops' morale meant that female nurses moved ever closer to the front line and were seen more and more as essential to the war effort. Furthermore, as the only female officers available for socialising, they were very much in demand. The medical officers needed to stop considering nursing staff as their servants and to treat them as equals if they wanted any of the attention for themselves. This necessarily altered the nurses' relationships with doctors.

Nursing sisters and medical officers

Attitudes towards the mixing of nursing and medical staff were highly circumscribed in the late nineteenth and early twentieth centuries.[162] However, during the Second World War attitudes appear to have softened and depended much more upon the hospital and its senior staff than upon any absolute rules. June Hamilton, who trained at a West London hospital from 1943, said that medical students were barred from the nursing students and that if you were caught talking to one, 'it was bad luck'.[163] Elizabeth Morris, who trained at The London, Whitechapel from 1944, recalled that junior nurses were not allowed to look the consultants in the eye.[164] Yet Salter's memories of her training school at St Mary's Paddington in London were of much more mixing and socialising together, with nursing and medical staff receiving free tickets to attend West End shows and trips to Twickenham to watch the medics play rugby.[165] According to Kevin Brown, Miss Milne, the matron of St Mary's, decided to relax the fraternisation rules between nurses and medical staff during the war, arguing that 'if her nurses had to work with medical students, they should be allowed to play with them too'.[166] This attitude worked in favour of improved relations on active service overseas. When Salter arrived at her posting at Ramree Island in the Bay of Bengal several weeks after she was expected, she promptly bumped into a naval officer who had been a medical student at St Mary's. They were both looking for the colonel and, when they found him, he had also been at St Mary's.[167] Such associations enabled the smooth running of hospitals and, in Salter's case, meant that she was not re-posted.

Before Sister Leeming was posted to Palestine she spent six weeks at Tidworth, a country mansion in the South of England. Apart from shopping trips and preparations for overseas service, 'We were also able to meet our M.O.'s who were mobilised in some distant place and parties were arranged to make our acquaintance.'[168] Relationships between medical officers and nursing sisters are discussed across all of the personal testimonies. Although some of the older medical staff treated the nurses in a more paternalistic manner, in the main, the testimonies describe congenial and respectful friendships. Dorothy Bartlett's memoir recalled a dinner at which the nurses and doctors were seated together, which she remarked made for interesting conversation because 'all the nurses seemed to have been placed next to the doctors or surgeons whose patients they were nursing'.[169] Whilst nursing sisters were likely to want to highlight developing collegiality in their testimonies, discussions of these friendships can also be found in recollections written by the doctors. McDonald wrote of his admiration for the sisters and the matrons, describing Miss Pike, the Principal Matron for Cairo, as a 'very alert and sensible person'.[170] Furthermore, he clearly saw the nursing sisters as social equals, as he and his MO colleagues spent much of their leisure time mixing with nursing sisters, especially playing bridge.[171] Such incidences would not only have broken professional and gender boundaries, but also enabled the two professions to learn more about each other's work. Significantly, the respect and friendship between McDonald and the nursing sisters of his unit extended into their professional lives; the matron of the unit, Miss Woolerton was present at the daily conference in McDonald's office along with his four medical colleagues.

Conclusion

The nursing sisters of the Second World War considered their presence in war zones as critical to the clinical encounter and the recovery of men. First, in the absence of strict hierarchies and in an environment in which the needs of the soldier as part of the machine of war were paramount, nursing sisters developed their use of self as part of the corporeal armoury of their work. Second, they developed a confidence in their use of humour to encourage recovery and to alleviate pain and promote well-being. Third, they used their newly formed, more collaborative relationships with medical staff to create greater autonomy of practice.

The use of self as an ideological tool of European femaleness and a way of encouraging continuation with fighting is more complex and creates a layer of ambiguity for the modern reader. These difficulties are partly related to mid-twentieth-century ideas of race and are partly to do with gender and the place and worth of women in society. Nevertheless, whether the nurses wholly accepted these notions, or whether it was a pragmatic recognition based on a desire to be on active service alongside fighting men, their personal testimonies do suggest an appreciation of their worth as being related to their gender and, to a lesser extent, their European ethnicity. As often the only female officers in far-flung war zones, overseas duty offered nurses new opportunities for social freedom. The negotiations based on gender, and sometimes crossing class boundaries, worked to the benefit of both men and women. However, they also had an additional benefit for nurses' professional standing. If their medical officers had continued to consider them as 'servants of the hospital' they, the doctors, would have lost out on valuable female company. In developing friendships, they also created a sense of collegiality that played into the professional environment and increased their understanding and respect of the nurses' clinical and recovery skills. These renegotiated relationships enabled a more fluid set of professional boundaries and a greater sense of trust. Nurses and doctors developed new therapeutic methods to recover men together, as colleagues bound by the exigencies of a highly mobile and technological war. It is these extended, expanded and new nursing roles that will be examined in the following chapter.

Notes

1 Agnes Kathleen Dunbar Morgan, 'My dearest mother', letter 87 (September 1944), CMF, 2, IWM Documents 16686.

2 Penny Starns, *Nurses at War: Women on the Frontline, 1939–45* (Stroud: Sutton Publishing, 2000), 37.

3 Morgan, letter 50, 'Obeying our General's orders'; Brenda McBryde, *Quiet Heroines: Nurses of the Second World War* (London: Chatto and Windus, 1985), 126. See also the various quotations in Crew, 'The Army medical services', from medical military men on the value of having female nurses in forward areas. F.A.E. Crew, 'The Army medical services', in Arthur Salusbury MacNalty and W. Franklin Mellor (eds), *Medical Services in War: The Principal Medical Lessons of the Second World War* (London: HMSO, 1968), 77–81. It should be noted that not all the quotations provided do support the front-line posting of nursing sisters.

4 Marsha L. Burris, *Paradox of Professionalism: American Nurses in World War II* (Charlotte: Spiral Publications, 2007), 96.
5 Pamela Bright, *Life in Our Hands: Nursing Sister's War Experiences* (London: Pan Books, 1955), 90.
6 The acknowledgement of gender as critical to the opportunities for women in war is explored by a number of historians in relation to work of all types. Women were never able to be simply workers, but always women workers, thus their femaleness was always more important than maleness for the men.
7 Cynthia Toman, *An Officer and a Lady: Canadian Military Nursing and the Second World War* (Vancouver: University of British Columbia Press, 2007), 100.
8 Toman, *An Officer and a Lady*, 10.
9 Barbara Caine, *English Feminism, 1780–1980* (Oxford: Oxford University Press, 2001), 176.
10 This performance of arch-femininity can be seen most coherently in Juliette Pattinson's work on women of the SOE negotiating their position as agents engaged in 'para-military' activity. Juliette Pattinson, '"Playing the daft lassie with them": Gender, captivity and the Special Operations Executive during the Second World War', *European Review of History* 13, 2 (2006): 276. See also Louise Willmot, 'Women and resistance', in Gilly Carr, Paul Sanders and Louise Willmot (eds), *Protest, Defiance and Resistance in the Channel Islands: German Occupation, 1940–45* (London: Bloomsbury, 2014).
11 Lucy Noakes, *Women in the British Army: War and the Gentle Sex, 1907–1948* (London: Routledge, Kindle edition, 2006), loc. 127.
12 Adrian Bingham, 'Enfranchisement, feminism and the modern woman: Debates in the British popular press, 1918–1939', in Julie V. Gottlieb and Richard Toye (eds), *The Aftermath of Suffrage: Women, Gender, and Politics in Britain 1918–1945* (Basingstoke: Palgrave Macmillan, 2013), 101.
13 Beth Linker, *War's Waste: Rehabilitation in World War I America* (Chicago: University of Chicago Press, 2011).
14 The origins of the concept of 'use of self' are found in nurse theorists' work on the therapeutic engagement of nurses with their patients. North American nurse-theorists Joyce Travelbee and Virginia Henderson and British nurse Richard McMahon argue that it is the nurse–patient relationship that is at the centre of their therapeutic engagement; that 'being with' the patient can make the difference. As Travelbee argued, the idea of the 'therapeutic use of self' is central to the nurse's engagement with their patient. Whilst these ideas were articulated after the Second World War, the chapter maintains that nurses in that conflict were aware that their presence and use of their 'nursing and female-selves', supported the healing and recovery of their soldier-patients. Joyce Travelbee, *Interpersonal Aspects of Nursing* (Philadelphia, PA: F.A. Davis, 1971); Virginia Henderson, *The Nature of*

Nursing: Reflections after 25 Years (New York: National League for Nursing Press, 1991), 24; Richard McMahon, 'Therapeutic nursing: Theory, issues and practice', in Richard McMahon and Alan Pearson, *Nursing as Therapy* (Cheltenham: Stanley Thornes, 1998), 6.

15 See, for example, Sheryl Nestel, '(Ad)ministering angels: Colonial Nursing and the extension of empire in Africa', *Journal of Medical Humanities* 19, 4 (1998): 257–77; Christina Twomey, '"Double displacement": Western nurses return home from Japanese internment camps in Second World War', *Gender and History* 21, 3 (2009): 670–84; Roland Sintos Coloma, '"White gazes, brown breasts": Imperial feminism and disciplining desires and bodies in colonial encounters', *Paedagogica Historica: International Journal of the History of Education* 48, 2 (2012): 243–61; Angharad Fletcher, 'Sisters behind the wire: Reappraising Australian military nursing and internment in the Pacific during World War II', *Medical History* 55 (2011): 419–24; Jessica Howell, Anne Marie Rafferty, Rosemary Wall and Anna Snaith, 'Nursing the tropics: Nurses as agents of imperial hygiene,' *Journal of Public Health* 35, 2 (2013): 338–41.

16 Emma Newlands, *Civilians into Soldiers: War, the Body and British Army Recruits, 1939–45* (Manchester: Manchester University Press, 2014), 146 .

17 Deebs Canning, John P. Rosenberg and Patsy Yates, 'Therapeutic relationships in specialist palliative care nursing practice', *International Journal of Palliative Nursing* 13, 5 (2007): 222–9.

18 Kara Dixon Vuic, *Officer, Nurse, Woman: The Army Nurse Corps in the Vietnam War* (Baltimore, MD: Johns Hopkins University Press, 2010, Kindle edition), loc. 146; Charlotte Dale, 'The social exploits and behaviour of nurses during the Anglo-Boer War, 1899–1902', in Helen Sweet and Sue Hawkins (eds), *Colonial Caring: A History of Colonial and Post-Colonial Nursing* (Manchester: Manchester University Press, 2015).

19 H.E. Whittingham, 'D.G.M.S. suggests the following reply to Dr Henderson's criticisms', MED/HIST/16: Items of historical interest, years 1940–41. Princess Mary's Royal Air Force Nursing Service Archive.

20 Maureen Honey, *Creating Rosie the Riveter: Class, Gender, and Propaganda during World War II* (Amherst, MA: University of Massachusetts Press, 1984), 202.

21 Mary Morris, *A Very Private Diary* (7 October, 1945), 265, IWM Documents 4850; Mary Morris, *A Very Private Diary: A Nurse in Wartime*, ed. Carol Acton (London: Weidenfeld and Nicolson, 2014), 265. For a wider discussion of Morris's marriage to an English officer, see Carol Acton, '"Stepping into history": Reading the Second World War through Irish women's diaries', *Irish Studies Review* 18, 1 (2010): 39–56.

22 Yasmin Khan, 'Sex in an imperial war zone: Transnational encounters in Second World War India', *History Workshop Journal* 73 (2012): 250.

23 Penny Summerfield, *Reconstructing Women's Wartime Lives: Discourse*

and Subjectivity in Oral Histories of the Second World War* (Manchester: Manchester University Press, 1998), 13.

24 Summerfield, *Reconstructing Women's Wartime Lives*, 14.

25 Cynthia Enloe, *Does Khaki Become You? The Militarization of Women's Lives* (London: Pandora, 1988), 213.

26 Enloe, *Does Khaki Become You?*, 106.

27 Morgan, 'My dearest mums', letter 55 (July 1943), MEF, 1.

28 Morgan, 'My dearest mums', letter 55 (July 1943), MEF, 2.

29 Scrub typhus had been differentiated from its rickettsial disease 'cousin' in the 1930s and research into it was accelerated during the 1939–45 conflict in response to the frequent epidemics in North Burma. According to Cornelius B. Philip, principal entomologist with the US Public Health Service in an article in 1948, 'the Americans' total of 695 cases for the entire campaign in that area, was exceeded by British casualties in each of 4 consecutive months, August to November inclusive, 1944, particularly along the Imphal jungle tracks and in the Kabaw and Chindwin Valleys to the east, including foci of major consequence in those areas'. One single battalion of the 2nd West Yorks had an infection rate of 18% in two months and a mortality of 5% of their total strength. Cornelius B. Philip, 'Tsutsugamushi disease (scrub typhus) in World War II', *The Journal of Parasitology* 34, 3 (1948): 169. From Salter's description, it appears that it was into this epidemic that she and her colleagues were sent. What is not known it whether it was the 2nd West Yorks that they nursed. Penny Salter, 'Long ago and far away: A distant memory': A diary, c. 1938–1970, 119–20, UKCHN archive, University of Manchester and IWM Documents 17649.

30 Salter, 'Long ago and far away', 119–20. The presence of nurses in the Burma campaign may have been a particular moment in their access to the front line. It is the only time that Mark Harrison mentions their presence as improving efficiency and boosting the morale of the combatant patients, 'despite some misgivings on the part of the male orderlies'. Mark Harrison, *Medicine and Victory: British Military Medicine in the Second World War* (Oxford: Oxford University Press, 2004), 219.

31 Salter, 'Long ago and far away', 122.

32 Salter, 'Long ago and far away', 122–3.

33 According to Kara Dixon Vuic, even in the mid-1960s, during the Vietnam War, recruitment campaigns for military nursing used the femininity of the nurse rather than her clinical skills as the method of patient healing. Kara Dixon Vuic, '"Officer, nurse, woman": Army Nurse Corps recruitment for the Vietnam War', *Nursing History Review* 14 (2006): 135.

34 Christine E. Hallett, *Containing Trauma: Nursing Work in the First World War* (Manchester: Manchester University Press, 2009), 158.

35 Santanu Das, *Touch and Intimacy in First World War Literature* (Cambridge: Cambridge University Press, 2005), 188.

36 Christine E. Hallett, '"This fiendish mode of warfare": Nursing the victims of gas poisoning in the First World War', in Jane Brooks and Christine E. Hallett (eds), *One Hundred Years of Wartime Nursing Practices, 1854–1953* (Manchester: Manchester University Press, 2015), 82.
37 McBryde, *Quiet Heroines*, 126.
38 Anonymous, 'Frontline Females', BBC Radio 4, 11 April 1998, British Library Sound Archive H9872/2.
39 Noakes, *Women in the British Army*, 1.
40 Noakes, *Women in the British Army*, 7. See John Laffin, 'Epilogue', *Women in Battle* (London: Abelard-Schuman, 1967), 184–5.
41 Morris, 'The diary of a wartime nurse' (19 June 1944), 94; Morris, *A Very Private Diary*, 83.
42 Iris Bower, 'From Normandy to the Baltic' (1985), 11, Princess Mary's Royal Air Force Nursing Service Archive.
43 Canadian Nursing Sister Nicholson remarked to Cynthia Toman in her oral history that the troops were horrified when the nurses landed with them at Sicily, but the nurses thought it was all rather exciting. Toman, *An Officer and a Lady*, 78.
44 Harrison, *Medicine and Victory*, 33.
45 George Feggetter, 'Diary of an R.A.M.C. surgeon at war, 1942–1946', 37, Wellcome Library, London, RAMC 1776.
46 Jessie Sarah Catherine Wilson, 'We also served', 19, UKCHN Archive, University of Manchester.
47 Evelyn Alma Cottrell, Spears Unit, reel 3. Oral history interview by Lyn E. Smith, 9 July 1990, IWM interview 12180.
48 Cottrell, reel 3, 9 July 1990.
49 Elsie Driver, 'Dear Miss Soutar' (9 July 1944), MMM QARANC uncatalogued archive.
50 Jean Bowden, *Grey Touched with Scarlet: The War Experiences of Army Nursing Sisters* (London: Robert Hale, 1959),142. In the correspondence with Miss Soutar, Driver does not mention the involvement of the matron, and her description of the soldiers seeing the nurses ashore is slightly different: 'We were I must admit, highly gratified when the troops showed such amazement and stood aghast, saying, "Golly, Sisters!!" and cheered us heartily'. Driver, 'Dear Miss Soutar'.
51 Catherine M. Butland, 'Army Sisters in Battledress or the Chosen Few or Follow Fate', 25, MMM QARANC/PE/1/74/BUTL Box 8.
52 Butland, 'Army Sisters in Battledress', 37; Wilson, 'We also served', 20.
53 Margarete Sandelowski, *Devices and Desires: Gender, Technology and American Nursing* (Chapel Hill, NC: University of North Carolina Press, 2000), 45.
54 Anonymous, 'In Step with the QAs. 1. – An officer writes to his wife from the Anzio beachhead', *The Nursing Times* 40, 32 (5 August 1944): 538.

55 Patricia Moody, 'My darling mums' (4 August 1943), 1, Royal College of Nursing (RCN) Archives, Edinburgh.
56 Francie E. Brown, 'My dearest Win and Moll', 59th British General Hospital, CMF (4 August 1944), IWM Documents 12472.
57 Morris, 'The diary of a wartime nurse' (19 December 1944), 163; Morris, *A Very Private Diary*, 142.
58 Butland, 'Army Sisters in Battledress', 74; Bower, 'From Normandy to the Baltic', 2.
59 L.K. Allen, 'A nursing sister's desert experience with the 8th Army', MMM QARANC uncatalogued archive.
60 Anonymous Sister, 'The Anzio beachhead', MMM QARANC uncatalogued archive, CMF file.
61 Butland, 'Army Sisters in Battledress', 47.
62 American officer, 99th General Hospital, B.N.A.F., MMM QARANC uncatalogued archive, British North Africa Campaign.
63 A.A. Nicol, *My Moving Tent: Diary of a Desert Rat* (Edinburgh: Pentland Press, 1994), 169.
64 Toman, *An Officer and a Lady*, 137. J.R. McDonald's diary is replete with high praise for the vast majority of nurses with whom he worked. J.R. McDonald (RAMC), 'A doctor goes to war', Wellcome Library, London, RAMC 944. Colonel C.R. Croft, RAMC, who was the O.C. for the desert hospital at which Sister Catherine Butland was the sister-in-charge, described her as 'an ideal type for a field unit and understands the requirements'. C.R. Croft, 'War diary, Alexandria, Egypt, No. 1 Mobile Military Hospital' (November 1942), TNA Medical Diaries, No. 1 Gen Hospital, WO 177/1093.
65 Feggetter, 'Diary of an R.A.M.C. surgeon at war', 37.
66 The nature of nursing as an art is discussed by Hallett, who identifies the artistry of nursing both in the engagement in fundamental nursing care and also in the improvisations that make patients feel better. Hallett, *Containing Trauma*, 13–15, 158. The complexity for nursing is that it may be an art, but in order to gain recognition and maintain itself next to the medical profession, it also demands that it is seen as a science. However, it seems that, despite this movement, it was the art of nursing that set it apart from the procedural, but no less considerate care of the orderly. Jane Brooks and Christine E. Hallett, 'Introduction: The practice of nursing and the exigencies of war', in Jane Brooks and Christine E. Hallett (eds), *One Hundred Years of Wartime Nursing Practices, 1854–1953* (Manchester: Manchester University Press, 2015), 6.
67 G.Q. Hunt, Lieutenant-Colonel, Grenadier Guards, 'Dear Sir' (11 May 1943). Letter to the Officer Commanding, General Hospital, M.E.F., MMM QARANC uncatalogued archive.
68 David Emery, 'Dear Sister Butland' (15 September 1945), MMM QARANC uncatalogued archive, MEF memoirs.

69 Feggetter, 'Diary of an R.A.M.C. surgeon at war', 37.
70 P.M. Dyer, 'When life was grey and scarlet: A recollection of life as an Army Nursing Sister', 22, MMM QARANC/PE/1/151/DYER Box 8.
71 Mary Anne Lagmay Tanay, Julia Roberts and Emma Ream, 'Humour in adult cancer care: A concept analysis', *Journal of Advanced Nursing* 69, 9 (2012): 2137.
72 Marion Cash, oral history interview via telephone by Jane Brooks, 23 October 2013.
73 Jean Clarke, oral history interview via telephone by Jane Brooks, 20 November 2013.
74 Ana Carden-Coyne, *The Politics of Wounds: Military Patients and Medical Power in the First World War* (Oxford: Oxford University Press, 2014), 321.
75 Cheryl Tatano Beck, 'Humor in nursing practice: A phenomenological study', *International Journal of Nursing Studies* 34, 5 (1997): 349; M. Greenberg, 'Therapeutic play: Developing humor in the nurse-patient relationship', *Journal of the New York State Nurses Association* 34, 1 (2003): 27.
76 Greenberg, 'Therapeutic play'; Ann D. Sumners, 'Professional nurses attitudes towards humour', *Journal of Advanced Nursing* 15 (1999): 200; Paivi Astedt-Kurki and Arja Isola, 'Humour between nurses and patient, and among staff: Analysis of nurses' diaries', *Journal of Advanced Nursing* 35, 3 (2001): 452.
77 Anonymous Sister, 'The Anzio beachhead'.
78 Morgan, 'My dearest mums', letter 61 (September 1943), CMF, 1.
79 Morris, 'The diary of a wartime nurse' (4 July 1944); Morris, *A Very Private Diary*, 102.
80 Morris, 'The diary of a wartime nurse' (2 July 1944); Morris, *A Very Private Diary*, 101.
81 Morris, 'The diary of a wartime nurse' (29 June 1944); Morris, *A Very Private Diary*, 101.
82 Mary Bond, *Wartime Experiences from the Midnight Sun to Belsen* (Cardigan: E.L. Jones and Son, 1994), 41.
83 Bower, 'From Normandy to the Baltic', 59.
84 Carden-Coyne, *The Politics of Wounds*, 183.
85 Sylvia Skimming, *Sand in My Shoes: The Tale of a Red Cross Welfare Officer with British Hospitals Overseas in the Second World War* (Edinburgh: Oliver and Boyd, 1948), 26.
86 Roberta Love Tayloe, *Combat Nurse: A Journal of World War II* (Santa Barbara, CA: Fithian Press, 1988), 46.
87 Betty C. Parkin, *Desert Nurse: A World War II Memoir* (London: Robert Hale, 1990), 92.
88 Morgan, 'My dearest mums', letter 85 (August 1944), CMF, 2.
89 Wilson, 'We also served'.
90 McBryde, *Quiet Heroines*, 127.

91 Ann Radloff, 'Going to Gooseberry Beach: Travels and adventures of a nursing sister', 16, IWM Documents 147.
92 Sumners, 'Professional nurses attitudes towards humour', 197.
93 Newlands, *Civilians into Soldiers*.
94 Butland, 'Army Sisters in Battledress'.
95 Anonymous, 'Topical notes – Normandy broadcast', *The Nursing Times* (1 July 1944): 430.
96 Emily Soper, oral history interview via telephone by Jane Brooks, 6 September 2013, UKCHN Archive, University of Manchester.
97 Butland, 'Army Sisters in Battledress', 74.
98 Eric Taylor, *Women Who Went to War, 1938–46* (London: Robert Hale, 1988), 127.
99 Radloff, 'Going to Gooseberry Beach', 17.
100 McBryde, *Quiet Heroines*, 127
101 Anonymous, 'December 1939–October 1942', 3, MMM QARANC uncatalogued archive.
102 Acting matron, 'A hospital ship at Tobruk, December 1941 to March 1942', in Ada Harrison (ed.), *Grey and Scarlet: Letters from the War Areas by Army Sisters on Active Service* (London: Hodder and Stoughton, 1944), 109.
103 Vera Jones, *A Time to Remember: A Record of Nursing Experiences, Impressions and Travels During World War II Contained in Letters Sent Home from The East* (London: Athena Press, 2005), 24.
104 Anonymous, 'Middle East and the hospital at Tobruk, December 1939–October 1942', MMM QARANC uncatalogued archive.
105 Anonymous, 'Dear Miss Wilkinson, H.M. Hospital Ship, Dorsetshire' (28 June 1941), MMM QARANC uncatalogued archive.
106 Salter, 'Long ago and far away', 114–15.
107 Morgan, 'My dearest mother', letter 23 (written and sent at a much later date for reasons of security), 1.
108 Betty Evans, oral history interview by Jane Brooks via telephone, 10 January 2014, UKCHN Archive, University of Manchester.
109 Morgan, letter 50, 'Obeying our General's orders', 1.
110 Salter, 'Long ago and far away', 62.
111 Wilson, 'We also served', 15.
112 Morris, 'The diary of a wartime nurse' (21 June 1944), 105; Morris, *A Very Private Diary*, 90.
113 Christina Twomey, 'Australian nurse POWs: Gender, war and captivity', *Australian Historical Studies* 36, 124 (204): 255–74.
114 John Costello, *Love, Sex and War: Changing Values, 1939–45* (London: Collins, 1985); Paul Fussell, *Wartime: Understanding and Behavior in the Second World War* (New York: Oxford University Press, 1989), 96–114; Gerard J. DeGroot, '"Lipstick on her nipples, cordite in her hair": Sex and

romance among British servicewomen during the Second World War', in Gerard J. DeGroot and Corinna Peniston-Bird, *A Soldier and a Woman* (Abingdon: Taylor and Francis, 2014).

115 Carden-Coyne, *The Politics of Wounds*, 245.

116 Christine E. Hallett, *Nurse Writers of the Great War* (Manchester: Manchester University Press, 2016), 212.

117 Costello, *Love, Sex and War: Changing Values*, 91.

118 Carden-Coyne, *The Politics of Wounds*, 191.

119 Hallett, *Containing Trauma*, 178.

120 Nell Jarrett, 'Diary of her desert experiences, 21 June 1942–13 January 1943' (30 July 1942).

121 Margaret Parkes, oral history interview by Jane Brooks at her home in the North West of England, 12 December 2012, UKCHN Archive, University of Manchester.

122 Emily Mayhew, *The Reconstruction of Warriors: Archibald McIndoe, The Royal Air Force and the Guinea Pig Club* (Barnsley: Greenhill Books, 2010, Kindle edition); Julie Anderson, *War, Disability and Rehabilitation in Britain: 'Soul of a Nation'* (Manchester: Manchester University Press, 2011); Liz Byrski, 'Emotional labour as war work: Women up close and personal with McIndoe's Guinea Pigs', *Women's History Review* 21, 3 (July 2012): 341–61.

123 Byrski, 'Emotional labour as war work', 353.

124 Anderson, *War, Disability and Rehabilitation in Britain*, 115.

125 According to Toman, several nurses that she interviewed were clear that there were some topics that they would not discuss. Key to this list were relationships between the medical and nursing staff on active service overseas, but which one nurse described as going 'a little bit beyond family'. Toman, *An Officer and a Lady*, 74.

126 LaVonne Telshaw Camp, *Lingering Fever: A World War II Nurse's Memoir* (Jefferson, NC: McFarland, 1997), 19.

127 The matter of British nurses being encouraged to attend dances was a novel departure for the Second World War. In the 1880s Catherine Grace Loch, the Superintendent of the Indian Army Nursing Service, forbade nurses from attending balls and dancing with officers, although Anne Summers states that this was over-ruled. Anne Summers, *Angels and Citizens: British Women as Military Nurses, 1854–1914* (Newbury: Threshold Press, 2000), 253. The prohibition against dancing was clearly reasserted in the First World War, as Christine Hallett provides an extensive quotation from the Matron-in-Chief Dame Maud McCarthy honouring the matrons for upholding the rule against dancing throughout the conflict and offering her permission that nurses should be allowed to dance to celebrate the Armistice. Christine E. Hallett, *Veiled Warriors: Allied Nurses of the First World War* (Oxford: Oxford University Press, 2014), 249.

128 Jane L. Forrest, 'Dear madam' (20 April 1943), MMM QARANC/PE/1/297/ Jones, collections and accounts 1943. Shaiba is in present-day Iraq – near Basra.

129 Jarrett, 'Diary of her desert experiences' (6 September 1942).

130 Betty Crisp, oral history interview via telephone by Jane Brooks, 13 January 2014. Crisp started nursing at the age of 16½ years at a cottage hospital on the south coast of England. UKCHN Archive University of Manchester.

131 Parkes, oral history interview, 12 December 2012.

132 For a full and detailed discssion on the discourse of morality and sexual propriety, see Sonya O. Rose, *Which People's War? National Identity and Citizenship in Britain, 1939–1945* (Oxford: Oxford University Press, Kindle edition, 2003).

133 Telshaw Camp, *Lingering Fever*, 90.

134 Salter, 'Long ago and far away', 125.

135 Parkes, oral history interview, 12 December 2012.

136 Catherine Hutchinson, 'My war and welcome to it', 22, IWM PP 02/36/1.

137 Barbara Collins, 'My dearest mummy and daddy', No. 51 General Hospital RAMC, Sierra Leone, British West Africa (26 August 1940), 2, UKCHN Archive, University of Manchester.

138 Howell et al., 'Nursing the tropics', 338.

139 Myra Valley, 'The training of "Agents of Empire": Educational and early career patterns for Scottish nurses of the Colonial and Overseas Nursing Associations, 1899–1939', *The Bulletin of the UK Association for the History of Nursing*, 3 (2014): 57–72.

140 Christina Twomey argues that although there was an increase in women professionals in colonial spaces, the vast majority of women in the tropics were colonial wives and daughters of male colonial officers. Furthermore, the Colonial Office encouraged marriage between Europeans in order to circumvent the possibility of 'sexual liaisons between British men and women of colour' (p. 672). For further discussions of the colonial project and Western women, see Sintos Coloma, 'White gazes, brown breasts', 245. For further discussion of American imperialism, see Winifred Connerton, 'American nurses in colonial settings', in Patricia D'Antonio, Julie A. Fairman and Jean C. Whelan (eds), *Routledge Handbook on the Global History of Nursing* (London: Routledge, 2013), 11–21.

141 Nestel, '(Ad)ministering angels', 258; Howell et al., 'Nursing the tropics', 338–41.

142 Jessica Howell, Anne Marie Rafferty and Anna Snaith, '(Author)ity abroad: The life writing of colonial nurses', *International Journal of Nursing Studies* 48 (2011): 1162.

143 Summers, *Angels and Citizens*, 150.

144 Lucy Bland, 'White women and men of colour: Miscegenation fears in Britain after the Great War,' *Gender and History* 17, 1 (April 2005): 29–61.

Bland argues that if sexual relations between white men and black women were 'unacceptable', those between black men and white women were 'totally reprehensible'. Bland, 'White women and men of colour', 31.

145 Kara Dixon Vuic, 'Wartime nursing and power', in Patricia D'Antonio, Julie A. Fairman and Jean C. Whelan (eds), *Routledge Handbook on the Global History of Nursing* (London: Routledge, 2013), 23.

146 Harrison, *Medicine and Victory*, 103.

147 Kevin Brown, *Fighting Fit: Medicine and War in the Twentieth Century* (Stroud: The History Press, 2008, Kindle edition), loc. 3494.

148 Khan, 'Sex in an imperial war zone', 245; Harrison, *Medicine and Victory*, 102.

149 Nestel, '(Ad)ministering angels', 258.

150 Sintos Coloma, 'White gazes, brown breasts', 250.

151 Wilson, 'We also served', 33.

152 John Cheetham, oral history interview by Jane Brooks, 8 September 2012. UKCHN Archive, University of Manchester. In his oral history interview, Cheetham, who had been in the tank corps in the desert, maintained that although when on leave in cities such as Cairo he did see nursing sisters, as an enlisted man, nursing sisters were 'out of bounds'.

153 Nell Jarrett's war diary remarks on the restrictions placed on them on the ship to Sierra Leone, 'we must not speak to the rough and licentious soldiery'. Jarrett, 'Diary of her desert experiences – England to Freetown' (2–13 June 1942).

154 Harrison, *Medicine and Victory*, 98.

155 Khan, 'Sex in an imperial war zone', 250.

156 Noakes, *Women in the British Army*, 35.

157 Fletcher, 'Sisters behind the wire', 420.

158 Summers, *Angels and Citizens*, 159.

159 Joanne Reilly, 'Cleaner, carer, and occasional dance partner? Writing women back into the liberation of Bergen-Belsen', in Jo Reilly, David Cesarani, Tony Kushner and Colin Richmond (eds), *Belsen in History and Memory* (London: Frank Cass, 1997), 156. Reilly in particular decries the 'glib' use of the word 'sacrifice', intoned in a narrative which, she argues, denies women's war efforts.

160 Salter, 'Long ago and far away', 124.

161 Radloff, 'Going to Gooseberry Beach', 23.

162 Anne Marie Rafferty, *The Politics of Nursing Knowledge* (London: Routledge, 1996), 29; Sue Hawkins, *Nursing and Women's Labour in the Nineteenth Century: The Quest for Independence* (London: Routledge, 2010), 25.

163 June Hamilton, oral history interview by Jane Brooks at her home in the south of England, 19 October 2011, UKCHN Archive University of Manchester.

164 Elizabeth Morris, oral history interview via telephone by Jane Brooks,

8 October 2013, UKCHN Archive University of Manchester. It is acknowledged that the position of consultants was quite different to that of all other professionals in the hospital. As honorary physicians and surgeons they gave their time in voluntary hospitals for free and were therefore treated with much greater deference. According to Mayhew, for example, McIndoe was known as either 'The Boss' or 'God' at East Grinstead. Mayhew, *The Reconstruction of Warriors*, loc. 1162.

165 Salter, 'Long ago and far away', 7.

166 Brown, *Fighting Fit*, loc. 4295.

167 Salter, 'Long ago and far away', 131.

168 E.M. Leeming, 'My war years, 1939–1945', 1, Wellcome Library, London, PP/LEE.

169 Dorothy A. Bartlett, *Nurse in War* (London: P.R. Macmillan, 1961), 108.

170 McDonald, 'A doctor goes to war', 198.

171 McDonald, 'A doctor goes to war', 166. Bridge appears to have been a particularly popular pastime on active service overseas, with nurses' testimonies also identifying it as an activity enjoyed by medical and nursing staff. Anonymous, 'In step with the QAs. 9. – Hospital ship (part II)', *The Nursing Times* (7 October 1944): 698.

4

Negotiating the boundaries of nursing practice

> Captain Johnson, the dental officer, a quiet man, spoke next. 'Treat for shock. Pick out any loose teeth and bits of bone then put a stitch through the tongue and tie it to a button on his jacket before you send him down the line on a stretcher'. His audience winced. Civvy nursing was never like this. These notes were probably intended for medical officers originally but they startled us into thinking objectively about the kind of nursing we might expect on active service.[1]

This quotation comes from Brenda McBryde's published memoir written nearly 50 years after the end of the Second World War. It is therefore prone both to relating the dramatic interventions required to engage a readership, and the nostalgia invoked by nurses when they considered their wartime lives. Nevertheless, it demonstrates the new surgical work that nurses expected to encounter as part of their overseas duties. Student nurses who trained between 1939 and 1945 cared for civilians injured by enemy bombing campaigns and combatants evacuated back to Britain from war zones. Thus, even before overseas posting, many nursing sisters had some experience of the horror of wounds caused by industrial weaponry. However, as suggested in the quotation above, the exigencies of active service, including the often limited access to medical officers, demanded innovative and rapid nursing responses to the life-threatening injuries of an increasingly technological war.[2]

Using surgical nursing in war as a 'case study' for developments in nursing practices and professional autonomy, the chapter examines the changes to the domain of their work by nursing sisters on active service overseas. The first section explores extensions to the nursing role, most particularly in the care of wounds and burns. Both of these areas of practice were part of the inventory of traditional nursing work, but the pressures of war demanded that all nurses should become adept at dealing with ever more complex treatments. Crucially for nursing sisters on active service, they were increasingly in charge of treatment regimes without medical supervision. The second section explores the expansion of nursing duties, those that had hitherto been the domain of medicine. These roles included the commencement and management of blood transfusions, surgical work and anaesthesia. The chapter's third section considers 'new work', the most critical of which was the administration and use of penicillin, although it is acknowledged that the utility of this drug went far beyond the treatment of surgical patients. This 'miracle drug' was one of the most important clinical developments for both medicine and nursing. Furthermore, because neither profession had previous experience with it, they needed to learn together, creating new lines of inter-professional relationships.

During the Second World War it was expected that women would become active citizens to help the war effort, but within the accepted gender constructions of femininity,[3] that is, maintaining a supportive and domestic sphere.[4] However, the importance of developing more collaborative working relationships between doctors and nurses was appreciated from the early months of the war, when the War Office ordered that RAMC medical officers and QAs attend gas courses together.[5] The placing of nurses and doctors in the same classroom as equals, even though it was not for clinical lectures, reveals the contradictory attitudes to men and women's participation in war. The male authorities both wanted and did not want there to be equal gender relations. Female nurses may have been very much the subordinate gender and profession in civilian hospitals, but the proximity of living and working quarters in a war zone made the continuation of the hierarchy difficult. Learning non-clinical skills together could facilitate the team-work that would be needed to recover men for battle. For nurses as members of the military posted overseas, edicts about femininity were increasingly difficult to follow, and untenable in the face of the proliferation of complex injuries and the new technologies developed to treat them.[6] As doctors on active service overseas established more collaborative relationships with nursing sisters outside the hospital wards and witnessed their work and apparent capabilities within those wards, they learnt to trust nurses to take on more complex work with less supervision and direction.

Shifting work and gender boundaries

As nurses extended and expanded their work beyond the 'normal' remit of nursing practice,[7] the gender and professional boundaries between medicine and nursing blurred. On active service overseas nurses increasingly 'stood in' for their medical colleagues as the exigencies of war demanded. One sister, part of the BEF evacuating Marseilles in June 1940, wrote that the colonel of her unit asked her about the medical fitness or otherwise of the patients: 'He said he could not find the M.O. to ask him. I gave my opinion.'[8] Sister Mary Morris's diary states that she and her colleagues, 'examined each man, carefully, referring any urgent cases to Col. Cordwell'.[9] Others prescribed and administered pain relief without a medical officer.[10] Sister Betty Parkin recalled passing a naso-gastric tube for a doctor when he was unable to do so.[11] Sister Angela Bolton maintained that 'The medical officers and sisters worked much more as a team than they did in hospitals back home. The unquestioning reverent obedience to doctors that had been instilled into us when we had been training had changed to an easy comradeship that made life pleasanter and more productive of ideas for the patients' welfare.'[12] Others wrote of 'rank [being] barely recognised'[13] and doctors helping the nurses on the ward as they created order out of the chaos of convoys.[14] Yet nursing sisters did not experience this new confidence without some hostility; not all relations in the field were harmonious. Sister Helen Luker experienced difficulties with the medical staff on the HMS *Dorsetshire*, both clinically and professionally. On 7 November 1940 she complains that 'Col Ward demands tea at 4.30pm to my intense annoyance'.[15] Then, on 20 December 1940 she wrote:

> We are just cleaning up after the transfusion when Pte Hughes, a gunshot wound of arm in plaster [*sic*] has a secondary haemorrhage. I have great difficulty in calling Capt. Robertson and when he comes he's not very helpful. We give packets of morphine and pray hard. I go to Capt. R twice more, but he doesn't think fit to get up & help us, so I do what I think is best. But Garland + I are simply shaking with anxiety + there are lots of other ill patients as well.[16]

Parkin's irritation was reserved for a medical officer who would not even let the nurses organise the diets, something she felt was entirely the province of nurses and not doctors.[17] Hutchinson wrote of a particular doctor, who having ordered a nursing sister to give a drug intramuscularly that should have been administered intravenously (IV) let the sister take the blame for the blunder. When this medical officer then asked Hutchinson to give the drug IV, she refused, stating, 'No, I do not have to. I am a Registered Nurse, and if I do not consider I am qualified to give a drug intravenously, I am entitled to refuse. I hereby refuse.'[18] Sister Joan Nicolson recalled the debacle following her refusal to work with a doctor who, she felt, had been overly harsh to a very young soldier who had deserted: 'And so of course I was in grave trouble because it was considered insubordination and his rank was major and I was only a lieutenant.' She was hauled in front of the colonel commanding her unit and informed him that 'I believed we should be sanctuary for people brought in'.[19] Although clearly guilty of insubordination, she was not disciplined. More importantly, both her behaviour and that of Hutchinson demonstrate a strength of will and professional confidence despite official medical superiority.

During the First World War men did not always appreciate being ordered by women, especially if those orders involved painful and arduous treatment regimes.[20] Despite the 20-year gap, many men had not altered their attitudes significantly.[21] Nurses were not necessarily allowed to enjoy professional autonomy in the same way that men did. Just as the Army needed to rely on the self-control of soldiers in far-flung war zones where the lines of authority were fewer,[22] so nurses were enabled to be more autonomous in these theatres of war, but this autonomy was contingent on geography and the levels of medical officer cover.[23] The closer to home and civilisation, the fewer the opportunities for new ways of practice, something that would have a lasting effect in the aftermath of war. Despite these impediments to the new working practices of nursing sisters, they managed to develop their role in new and professionally legitimating ways.

The adoption of 'medical' tasks by nurses was not new and there had always been a body of nurses who had little use for the constraints of professional boundaries.[24] Where they saw a problem, they dealt with it.[25] As medical technologies became commonplace – such as the thermometer in the early twentieth century, the sphygmomanometer

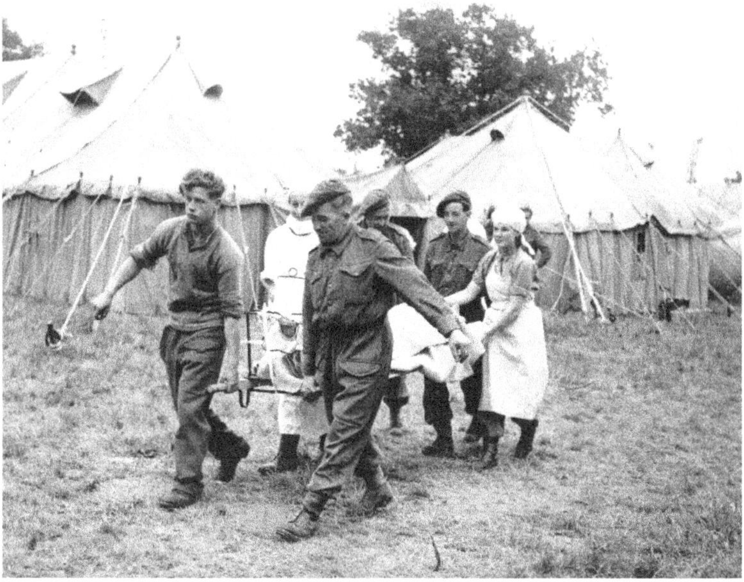

8 Italy. Sisters and RAMC orderlies carrying out a patient. This image reveals the collegiality between different members of the medical team. Such relationships were essential for successful patient care in active service conditions.

(the instrument used for taking blood pressures) and the monitoring of intravenous infusions in the inter-war period – doctors were pleased to hand over this now mundane work.[26] However, on active service overseas nurses were required not only to take over technologies from their medical colleagues[27] but also to develop skills with new technologies alongside doctors, thus shifting the balance from learning 'from' the medical profession to learning 'with' medical colleagues.

Extending nursing work

Wound care

The exigencies of war had a profound effect not only on those nurses who were posted overseas but also those nurses and probationers who were required to care for combatants on British soil after ill and injured soldiers were evacuated back to 'Blighty'.[28] Traditional hospital 'dressing rounds', as they were called, followed an ordered formula, with little room for individual decision making. In a hospital system where student nurses performed the majority of nursing work, such formulaic practice made perfect sense. Nurses needed to be able to care for patients with 'unconscious competence', in order to prevent accidental harm.[29] There were aspects of the dressing-round ritual that included some level of decision making, such as not beginning dressings until after the dust had settled following the daily cleaning regime. Changeable criteria that required skills in negotiating indeterminacy,[30] such as beginning with the cleanest wounds and leaving the most dirty or infected wounds till the end, thereby altering the organisation of the round, were not necessarily part of the process.[31] The onslaught of injured men from battle denied the hospital-ward dressing round its ritual. Nurses needed to develop more reactive nursing skills rapidly. Morris's experiences as a student following the evacuation of soldiers from Dunkirk were to provide excellent training for her overseas postings:

> As I entered the Casualty department, I was astounded to see so many wet, dirty and injured people there. Some were soldiers (I guessed they must be Dunkirk survivors), others were civilians … they were all laid out on stretchers on the floor, and most of our surgeons and physicians were there, assisted by several senior Sisters and Staff Nurses. I was given the job of removing dirty wet clothing, so that they could be examined by the doctors. Several men had their skin flayed by oil burns, a very painful condition, others were injured by bomb splinters, and some injured by machine gun fire from the air as they came across the Channel.[32]

Sister Penny Salter's recollections of the arrival of convoys from Dunkirk, when she was a student, invoke the same level of suffering. Like Morris, the work caring for the survivors would prepare her partly for the challenges that she would face when posted overseas:

> At 2.30 am we ran across the grounds and down the long cold and dreary corridors of Park Prewett Hospital meeting on the way the male orderlies, strangers to us, of whom we learned at a later date were volunteer pacifists who had been up all night helping with the evacuation of the hospital … on that May morning in 1940, the ambulances began to arrive, carrying the maimed, the lame and the blind. Many were on stretchers, others limping along supported by weary comrades clinging to them.

> Everything here was well organized, the teamwork between doctors and nursing staff was outstanding, not a moment was lost in dealing with the terrible injuries we had to face: foul, putrid festering wounds that stank to high heaven, sustained by men of remarkable courage.
>
> Our first task was to get them bathed and cleaned up before putting them to bed in to cool crisp sheets, but this was not easy as their feet was [*sic*] the problem. Their feet were in such a terrible state that even after soaking we had to cut their boots off.
>
> The stench of dried blood and gangrenous flesh was nauseating. I remember so well asking an orderly to stay with one of my patients for a short while as, so like many of my colleagues I went outside and was violently sick … the stench remained in my nostrils for days.[33]

These experiences as students may have prepared them for the smell and decay of war injuries, but the challenges of work on overseas postings stretched the Army nurses' expertise 'to capacity'.[34] On active service the limited access to medical staff, the severity of the injuries that required dressings, the sheer numbers of combatants arriving needing nursing care, the complexities of the wounds and the prolonged period between the wound being sustained and the access to a qualified nurse conspired to create the 'perfect storm' of work.[35] In a 1940 publication designed to prepare the nurse for war service, the work of the surgical nurse is described as, 'a strange experience … at the beginning they will often be shocked by the physical enormities that are inevitable in war as it is waged to-day'.[36]

Many of the complex wounds that nurses were required to dress on active service overseas would have been seen to by medical staff, or at least under supervision of a doctor in civilian practice. Bruce Dick, a consulting thoracic surgeon, wrote that war nurses would need 'resourcefulness in certain emergencies' that perhaps had hitherto not been necessary.[37] In his letter to *The Lancet*, John Elam maintained that nurses and other first-aid workers should all be trained in gas and air analgesia 'for the dressing of war wounds'.[38] Morris was clearly proud of the 'resourcefulness' of their surgical team in Normandy: 'Another new M.O. arrived here today. He is very pleasant but rather astonished by our unconventional methods of surgery and post operative [*sic*] nursing. We have all learned a great deal here, mainly by trial and error. Necessity has created a great deal of inventiveness.'[39]

In the wars of the twentieth century, hospitals could provide valuable respite for battle-exhausted soldiers, but the injuries sustained also created the need to perform what could seem like barbaric surgical interventions.[40] Nursing sisters knew that it was their 'meticulous care in regard to asepsis at all times, in spite of hectic rushes [which] may mean the difference of a man keeping or losing a limb'.[41] However, sometimes men arrived having had the amputation in the field, using brutal methods developed to prevent gangrene. In June1940, the *Nursing Times* informed its readers that in order to prevent gangrene spreading through the stump flap following amputation, 'a new and drastic form of amputation – known as a guillotine amputation – was introduced'.[42] In the desert war from late 1941, nurses were witnessing and writing about the damage that this method caused. One TANS sister wrote to Dame Katharine Jones expressing her distress over the 'Many limbs [that] had to be re-amputated as the first operation had been performed up in the front line C.C.S. by Greek M.O.s. The limb had been cut off, arteries tied and a dressing applied leaving a great raw wound that could never heal. It was very difficult to make the patients understand why they must have a second operation.'[43] It is unlikely that even as Matron-in-Chief, Jones was able to affect the decision to stop using the guillotine method, but, critically, nurses were gaining in confidence to question surgical practice. Furthermore, they needed to use all their skills to support their soldier-patients for future surgery.

The extension of nurses' work with war injuries thus gave rise to new demands for psychological care. It was of vital importance for nurses 'to gain the patient's confidence and co-operation' in order to provide life-saving and -affirming treatments.[44] Morris wrote in her diary of her concern for one lieutenant who had sustained an abdominal wound during the fighting at Arnhem in the autumn of 1944: 'Brian will be alright physically once the wound has healed but I think it will be a long time before he gets over the shock of Arnhem. Connie tells me that he has to be constantly sedated at night to stop him screaming in terror. He is only twenty-two years old.'[45] Sister Catherine Hutchinson's greatest sympathies lay with her patients who had colostomies. Medical authorities knew that in order for abdominal injuries to have any hope of healing, immediate surgery was needed, but this led to men being operated upon and then having days before any further treatment.[46] Many of Hutchinson's patients had sustained gunshot wounds to the abdomen and then had travelled by train through Italy to Naples before being admitted to her ward on HMS *Empire Clyde*:

> During these days – for days it was – rather than hours – some of them had not had their dressings (they had not got to the stage of bags yet) properly changed – just more padding added as the bandages became stained with faecal fluid. They bulged horrifically as if bearing a pillow over their abdomen. If the ship was in the Naples harbour they came direct to us exhausted, apprehensive and stinking ... I took note of such patients, knowing that I would have to struggle to undo the work of neglect … When all the dressings were off, a sorry state was revealed. Because most of them were recent casualties, the outpourings were mostly fluid or semi solid; the acidity in the fluid had excoriated the skin around the opening in a wide area, leaving most of the abdomen red and sore, with broken skin around the actual opening.[47]

Hutchinson's acknowledgement of the scale of her responsibility for the wounded men is tempered by her understandable dismay at their surgery and the realisation that she will need to do more than just care for the men's physical needs. Evidence of sporadic and occasionally successful performance of colostomies can be found from the eighteenth century. According to Dorothy Doughty, in one of the only historical essays on stoma surgery, by the twentieth century colostomies had become a realistic treatment option, although the products to support colostomy care were still in their infancy.[48] The horror of the colostomy was not lost on the nurses or medical staff. The narrative of the disgust that a stoma creates in people was exemplified in the 1956 propaganda film *The Feminine Touch*.[49] In the film, designed to improve recruitment and retention in the post-war nursing profession,[50] the character of the matron uses the tragedy of the colostomy to dispel any question as to the vital importance of the nurse's work in psychological as well as physical rehabilitation of the patient with a stoma. It is the nurse, the matron argues, and her response to the stoma that makes the difference to whether the patient can also accept the surgery. Even though Hutchinson maintained that she never had more than two colostomy patients at once,[51] the stench from dressings that had not been changed since the original operation in the claustrophobic atmosphere of a hospital ship would have increased the revulsion for all concerned. As the nursing sister in charge of the ward, Hutchinson's commitment to extending her nursing skills was paramount to recovering the men.

The new technologies of the Second World War created advanced weaponry that could maim and harm with extensive and devastating consequences. The medical services were challenged to respond rapidly and with the requisite skills to save life. Some of the worst examples of these assaults on the human body involved burning. Many nursing sisters had some experience of caring for burns and some had received special post-registration training. Brenda McBryde attended the burns course at Bangor that had been instituted in the wake of the terrible injuries that had been sustained by airmen in 1940 during the Battle of Britain.[52] Not all of the nursing sisters were so fortunate to receive specialist training prior to their overseas posting. All were shocked at the havoc that burns wreaked on their victims, whether from aircraft that went up in flames, burning oil as ships sank or being trapped in tanks.[53] The developments in burns treatments meant that nurses were confronted with new and constantly evolving therapeutic regimes to salvage their soldier-patients.

Burns

E.C. Davidson 'revolutionised' burns treatment in 1925 when he introduced tannic acid. By the beginning of the Second World War the use of tannic acid for burns had been standardised and it was believed that their treatment therefore would cause 'little difficulty'.[54] In July 1940, in an article examining the treatment of incendiary bomb burns, the advice from Dr R.G. Henderson was that tannic acid of a strength varying from 5 per cent to 20 per cent should be either sprayed or dabbed with gauze onto the burn. If this was then followed by an application of 10 per cent silver nitrate solution, a protective crust would be formed.[55] By November of that year the *Nursing Mirror* was alerting its readers to the cessation of using tannic acid routinely for burns.[56] Nurses were alerted to the dangers of tannic acid in the treatment of third degree burns and those on the hands and face, because of the extensive scarring and contractions that it could cause.[57] Most nursing staff would not necessarily have been aware of the research into the treatment of burns with tannic acid, but, even as a junior probationer, Morris would bear witness to the damage that it created when used on the hands and face:

> Private Brian M. is one of the most severely burned. He is about eighteen years old – my age. His face and hands have been sprayed with tannic acid, which has set into a hard black cement. His arms are propped up in front of him on a pillow, the fingers extended like claws and his naked body hangs loosely on straps just clear of the bed.[58]

Yet as nurses observed the catastrophe of burns, they were not always passive onlookers. Because all the methods of treating burns were dependent upon the nursing care,[59] their observations would enable them to support developments in burns care as the war continued. One anonymous sister in the Middle East noted that 'dyes, e.g. Triple dye treatment of burns was not a success in the topics'.[60] Another nursing sister was posted to Gibraltar between 1940 and 1942: 'I had ample opportunity of [*sic*] observing and comparing the merits of modern treatment for burns: tannic acid, triple dye, Vaseline and sulphonamide powder, saline baths and dressings, and I was much impressed by the excellent results obtained by enclosing limbs for several weeks in Plaster of Paris.'[61] Sister V. Shennan's extensive notes sent to Dame Katharine Jones in 1943 from the Middle East on the care of the burns patient and the complex arrangements for treatment regimens suggest the close involvement of nurses in decisions regarding the needs of the patient. For example, she identified the actions to be taken in the case of a reaction to blood transfusions, the protocols for dressings and contra-indications to sulphonamide 'emulsions'.[62]

By 1941 the treatment for burns had developed significantly, following knowledge gained in the first two years of the war. Wing Commander Stanford Cade of the RAF acknowledged the worth of tannic acid and its life-saving value in civilian life, but argued that the nature of 'Airman's burns' was such that its benefits were reduced.[63] Tulle gras dusted with sulphanilamide and kept moist with saline drips was now the treatment of choice for many burns. Where the burns affected limbs, jaconet or silk bags were recommended to retain the moisture and promote healing.[64] These new treatments were also less painful than tannic acid.[65] The alternative was the envelope or Bunyan method, named after John Bunyan, the surgeon who invented it. In 1942, Archibald McIndoe was advocating tannic acid and silver nitrate for non-functioning parts of the body, such as the back or abdomen.[66] However, for burns to the hands and face or in the case of third degree burns he argued for the use of sulphanilamide tulle gras moistened with saline, if possible in conjunction with saline baths.[67] Despite these new treatment options, the debates as to the relative harms and benefits of tannic acid and other regimens continued throughout the war. In her diary entry for 9 November 1944, Bolton wrote of a patient who was 'the worst case of burns I have seen out here, three-quarters of the skin surface being involved ... we badly need a breakthrough for burns'.[68] Despite the developments in burns care, even in the latter months of the war, the choices were limited and success rates not certain.

Like Morris and Salter, Sister Ann Radloff gained useful experience in caring for injured soldiers as a student nurse in Britain, including those who had been burnt. In her memoir, she recalled the archaic nature of tannic acid and other topical treatments and demonstrated a prescient understanding of the regimes for shock:

> The troopship Lancastria was bombed and sunk off Cherbourg. Very few of the survivors could walk – how can you when you have been covered in flaming oil? Those were the days of Tannic Acid (sometimes even cold tea leaves were used) for treatment of burns. And the Bunyan bag was an enormous cellophane container filled with saline into which charred limbs were inserted to be entirely surrounded by fluid. Corporal C. – 'Jock' – was an unrecognizable human hulk with a human soul. He had been enveloped in burning oil and as a living torch had jumped into the sea. Perhaps the salt water saved him but the oil was thick and cohesive and had burnt right through to the tissues. Jock had to be moved and turned – worst of all he sometimes had to be lifted onto a bedpan. The skin contracted and Jock was never free from pain unless mercifully drugged with morphine ... All severe burns cases suffered from dehydration which can be remedied by a saline drip, if, as in Jock's case the lips are too corroded and swollen and the tongue too painful for fluid to be given by mouth. But they could not find a vein in Jock's charred body. So Corporal C. died ...[69]

Others were luckier and the sea did in fact save them. Betty Evans, working as a student nurse in London during the Dunkirk evacuation, noted 'a terrific number of pilots baling with dreadful burns, baling out into the sea ... but the pilots were baling out into the flames and so had dreadful burns, but the ones who were in the water, because of the saline, their skin grafts did better'.[70] Sisters Geraldine Edge and Mary Johnstone were posted to the Hospital Carrier *Leinster*, from where they evacuated patients between Naples and Anzio. On one such trip they embarked 30 American sailors, all of whom had been burnt when their ship was torpedoed: 'hours of immersion in cold water seems a harsh method of dealing with such cases, but the effect of salt water on burns is found to be extraordinarily good and strangely enough the ensuing shock is less'. Although at least one did die, many survived.[71]

Too often, as Lt-Colonel Norman Logie (RAMC) wrote in *The Lancet* of his experience in caring for burns victims in the desert, there were no nurses. Although, as he maintained, the orderlies did what they could to support the healing of burns patients, 'they were not nurses and they were few in number'. They needed simple regimes that were not affected by the frequent dust storms and the need for lengthy evacuation journeys. He therefore recommended tannic acid and silver nitrate for burns, but not of the hands and face, which should be treated with tulle gras soaked in sulphanilamide.[72] However, he cautioned over the possible toxicity from contact of sulphanilamide with raw areas that could raise the blood concentration to a 'dangerous level'.[73] By 1944 penicillin was available for burns, thus theoretically rendering such concerns obsolete. Evans, who landed with the Second Front into France in 1944, recalled using penicillin in conjunction with tulle gras on the burns of men who had been trapped in tanks, but there were fears that penicillin would not be beneficial in all burns cases.[74]

Although tannic acid in conjunction with silver nitrate was an uncertain cure, according to Brigadier Philip Mitchiner, honorary surgeon to the king, it was useful as a first-aid measure in many burns, except those on the face and hands, and was particularly useful in preventing shock.[75] McIndoe wrote in the *Nursing Mirror* that 'the first and most important thing is the control of shock. This takes precedence over any form of local treatment, apart from the protection of the burn and the dusting on of sulphanilamide powder.' PMRAFNS Sister H.B. Woods also claimed precedence for the treatment of shock as the primary concern, followed by the prevention of infection.[76] Woods' dictum that these were the primary responsibilities for nurses in burns cases is critical, given their position in the overseas military medical service. She recommended the treatment of shock by warming the patient with electric blankets and hot-water bottles and then the administration of warm fluids orally, per rectum or intravenously[77] – work which would have been understood as nursing. Evans maintained that even in the summer of 1944 they had the 'medical staff putting up the drips',[78] yet many nurses had taken on IV therapy as part of their nursing role. The administration of IV plasma had become a nursing duty before the war, but the frequency of infusions and the lack of medical staff to monitor them on active service overseas meant that its place in the lexicon of nursing work increased. As the war raged around the nurses at the Anzio beachhead, one nurse wrote that: 'In the Post-Operative Ward it was unusual to find a patient who was not having either blood or plasma, and the care of the "drips" was one person's constant work.'[79] In an article to the *Nursing Mirror* on 2 September 1939, the day before war was declared, nurses were informed that their duty was: 'The care of the recipient, which will include the preparation of the site to be used … sterilising and the preparation of the necessary apparatus … the doctor … controls the flow when the apparatus cannot be adjusted and safely left without attendance.'[80] As the long years of the war progressed and realisation grew of the changing requirements that were being placed on the medical services, the roles of the nursing staff needed to expand to this challenge.

Expanded nursing work

Transforming transfusions

> Our Medical Office [*sic*] being so busy receiving patients could not always be present at admissions. This was to our advantage as we became well acquainted with the stethoscope and commenced to do our own investigations for diagnosis, to be checked later by the Medical Officer. Besides becoming quite adept at diagnosing we learned to do many treatments which we would not be allowed to do at home. What a great thrill I had at setting up my first blood transfusion.[81]

Whether in Britain or on active service overseas, when medical officers could not be spared to monitor blood transfusions, such work was passed to the nursing staff. Thus, by 1943, June Hamilton stated, even student nurses in Britain were monitoring the blood flow of a transfusion and it was accepted that the staff nurse would take action if the flow stopped. Only if the staff nurse could not start the flow again would the registrar be informed.[82] According to Margarete Sandelowski, the delegation of work because of the inconvenience of mundane activities to the medical profession maintained a strict hierarchy between professions and, by implication. gender.[83] Nurses' duties expanded into key positions in the resuscitation wards on active service overseas, work that was critical in restoring men with shock before surgery. The right of the medical staff to dictate that work had not altered. McBryde recalled the order: 'Quarter of morphia, Sister. Straight away. Two pints of blood, one of plasma.'[84] At times, nurses were simply unable to find a medical officer when the convoys arrived, and their willingness to start transfusions without medical supervision was paramount if men were to survive.[85] As Sister P.M. Dyer's quote above demonstrates, British nurses were excited rather than alarmed when war brought with it a range of new tasks, and did not necessarily view the delegation of the work as a sign of their subservience.

The limited access that British women had to the medical profession in the early years of the twentieth century meant that few considered it as a real option. This left nursing as the natural choice for those who wished to care for the sick and support the health of the community.[86] At least two of the nurses' testimonies used in this book identify that they had brothers who were either doctors or officers in the war, suggesting a gender rather than class split.[87] Whilst nurses were deferential to doctors, there is little evidence to suggest that they considered either themselves or the work that they did as subordinate to medicine. Even deference reduced as nurses gained the professional and personal confidence that came with active service.[88] Nor is there evidence that they saw the delegation of tasks previously considered 'medical' as an indication of their subordination. Rather, they greeted with enthusiasm the implication that they were now seen as worthy and capable colleagues; this perhaps especially when sometimes the nurses transfused patients and sometimes the medical staff did.[89] If work was interchangeable, it could not be subordinate.

During the First World War research into shock and haemorrhage led to developments in blood transfusions, but these involved highly complex and time-consuming techniques.[90] By 1918, although methods for storing whole blood had been developed, these were too late to be of benefit to most soldiers.[91] The understanding of blood grouping was embryonic and, according to Carden-Coyne, there were only a few units that had the expertise to carry out the process.[92] Furthermore, the instructions that most medical officers had been given in respect of the provision of blood transfusions were inadequate.[93] Given the potential dangers of the transfusion procedure, it required the active participation and supervision of medical staff, with the support of nursing sisters and orderlies. By the time of the Spanish Civil War, 'great strides' had been made in the storage and preservation of blood for transfusion, enabling nurses and doctors to treat shock quickly and with good effect. However, the technologies, still in their infancy, meant that medical and nursing staff continued to provide direct transfusions, sometimes acting as donors themselves. This created the additional hazard that often too much blood was taken from these essential workers, who then needed periods of rest and recuperation themselves.[94]

Cynthia Toman argues that as blood transfusion work was delegated to nurses in the Second World War, it lost its place as a prestigious medical technology and became simply another job for the nursing staff.[95] The delegation of medical tasks to nurses as the work becomes commonplace and mundane exemplifies Margaret and Patrice Higonnet's 'double helix' in which women are always subordinated and 'other'. When work is handed to women, not only is it because men no longer want it, but it is concurrently devalued because it now belongs to women.[96] However, this is perhaps too simplistic or rigid a way to understand the expansion of nursing work and the delegation of what was once medical work to nurses.[97]

The great changes in transfusion technology between the First and Second World Wars meant that far more people could benefit from blood transfusion therapy and the therapy itself was no longer experimental. Sister D.M. Long wrote of the life-saving benefits of rapid transfusion that could now be given with 'no fuss'.[98] Once blood transfusions became something from which people expected to benefit and did not carry the risks of experimental medicine, in order to prevent it being a dehumanising technology the apparatus needed a human buffer.[99] Thus the Second World War nurse not only made the technology possible but was the human face that enabled the patient to accept it.[100] That is not to argue that the work had not become mundane to the medical officers who wanted to pass it on, but that there were also positive reasons for nurses to take on such work. The reassignment of blood transfusion care was arguably a natural progression as it moved from an experimental procedure that demanded medical expertise in the First World War, to a procedure that demanded the close monitoring of both technology and patient, both of which came and continue to be part of nursing, rather than medicine. It was not only that the medical profession delegated what had become simple work to nurses, but that blood transfusion had now become nursing work because its nature had changed.

The organisation of the British Blood Transfusion Service in 1938, shortly after the Munich Treaty, was to give the British Army a significant advantage over all other nations.[101] It meant that safe, whole blood could be accessed quickly. The Americans had discovered in 1939 that unfiltered blood plasma was a useful substitute for whole blood, and continued to use it, often in place of whole blood. However, it was not as effective as whole blood in treating shock. On 5 October 1939, the Transfusion and Surgical Research Laboratory left for France. This laboratory was disbanded after the evacuation from Dunkirk in the summer of 1940, after which the British Transfusion Unit was established.[102] In 1941, whilst undertaking her training, Emily Soper was allocated to join her hospital's transfusion unit:

> We had a sister and staff nurse came from what was called the Civil Defence Unit and surprise, surprise, I was made their junior. So when the siren went off, we had to report to our, er, little quarters that were allotted to us, so we had to be ready, but fortunately again, we were not required to use our blood transfusion expertise on any casualties, but we were delegated to help our doctors, if they needed any help in the hospital.[103]

Importantly, with such a system in place in civilian practice, the military medical authorities were able to transfer knowledge rapidly into the field. By the spring of 1940, it was acknowledged that all medical officers, nurses and orderlies would have to understand the essentials of storing, preserving and administering blood transfusions for shock. It was no longer work for a few specialist units; the technology and clinical practice requirements meant that blood transfusions were transformed from a complex, medical task to essential therapy.[104] C.A. Wells, an honorary surgeon at the Royal Liverpool Hospital, wrote in the *Nursing Times* in July 1945 that 'first bottle of blood I ever saw in a refrigerator was in the Meath Hospital in Dublin in 1939, I do not care to think how many I have seen since then!'[105] In April 1942, a *Nursing Times* editorial reflected on wartime advances in medicine and surgery, commenting on the great change in the provision in blood transfusion: 'whereas before the war it would be two hours on average from the time the telephone rang in his [the doctor's] house to the time the needle was in the vein, to-day he could be starting the infusion within 20 minutes from the first tinkle of the bell'.[106]

In October 1944, Morris was working in a hospital set up in a convent near Louvain. Despite this not being particularly close to the front line, there was clearly a more collaborative way of working in which inter-professional expectations of practice were blurred. Thus, the nurses engaged in expanded areas of practice and the medical staff would help with the more nursing-type patient care of settling men into bed. They took convoy after convoy, some from CCSs near Nijmegen and others from a hospital near Arnhem:

> Some were given plasma at once, others blood transfusions as soon as we could identify the group (We have a small blood bank here) … Have just crawled off duty at 2 a.m. The patients are cleaned up, undressed (we had to cut off their clothing) and in bed. There are six blood transfusions and 13 blood plasmas 'on the go'. Hope Connie can manage for the rest of the night. She has two good orderlies.[107]

As the military medical services responded to the needs of a mobile war in which men could be treated much closer to the front, hospitals and CCSs were increasingly supported by independent blood transfusion units.[108] One nursing sister noted that 'Blood transfusion and resuscitation service are splendidly organised especially in the forward areas'. This was particularly vital, since 'Gun shot wounds of abdomen are received into warm beds, a blood transfusion given at once and treatment for shock carried out.'[109] Sister E.L. L'Estrainge also noted the importance of the blood transfusion unit running independently from theatre.[110] Given that all the casualties were exhausted and needed blood, this separate service could provide blood as necessary without removing the surgeon, theatre sister or

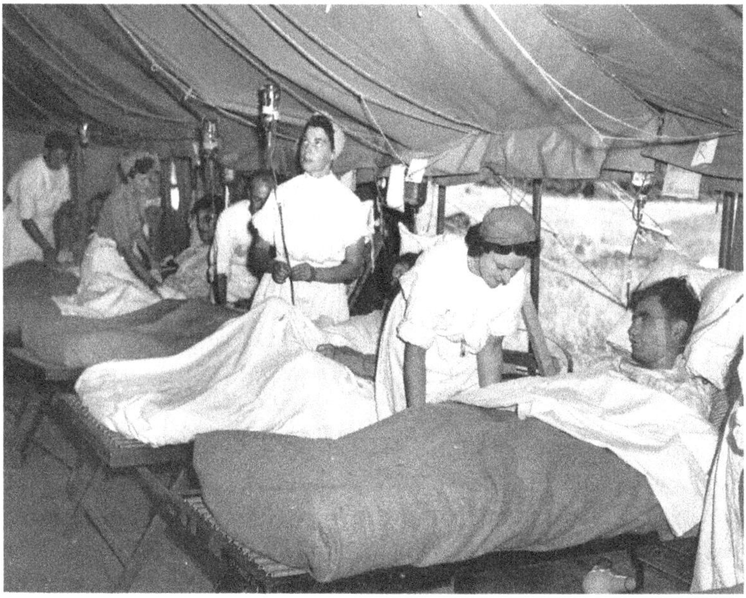

9 Nurses and patients in a field hospital. This image shows us the nurse's central role in blood transfusions. It is also worth noting the dramatic alterations in the uniform worn in comparison with the image of Nell Jarrett as a student nurse in figure 1. The nursing sister in this image of a field hospital in northern Europe is not restricted by either uniform or profession boundaries.

orderlies from the operating table. This was not the case in all situations. The hospital ship the *Llandovery Castle* collected its blood from Alexandria for each journey. The blood then became the responsibility of the surgeon, the trained orderly and the theatre sister.[111]

In whatever manner a particular blood transfusion system was organised on active service overseas, accountability was invariably cross-professional. The medical military authorities appreciated that 'blood work' was now an essential part of war medical services and needed support and collegiality to ensure that blood was stored and administered safely and efficiently. Unlike some other practices, blood work remained part of the lexicon of nursing duties post-war.[112] Alongside nurses' participation in ever more complex wound care, it was clearly not a cause of inter-professional angst. However, there were other roles that were handed to nurses only 'for the duration' and only because of the extreme challenges of the war. Possibly the most controversial expanded role was that of nurses in anaesthetics.[113]

The nurse-anaesthetist

Between 1940 and 1942 a series of letters, many verging on the vitriolic, appeared in the *British Medical Journal* in relation to nurse-anaesthetists. All were written by medical staff, none of whom appear to have been on active service overseas. On 28 September 1940, F.B. Parsons forwarded to the *British Medical Journal* a letter from medical staff of Addenbrooke's Hospital in Cambridge to the Association of Anaesthetists. In the letter they argued that 'with the outbreak of war five out of the eight honorary anaesthetists to the hospital were mobilised and left the district'.[114] Since that time, the hospital had relied on the remaining three and increasingly junior and inexperienced medical officers to undertake anaesthetic duties, whilst the numbers of patients within the hospital rose. This, they felt, was unsustainable. The answer was to train nurses 'who had held the post of sister in a ward or operating theatre' to give anaesthetics.[115] They would not supplant honorary anaesthetists, but would support the work of their colleagues in the operating theatres and, therefore, their patients.

The decision caused uproar. Nurses had been employed to act as anaesthetists by the British military on active service overseas in the First World War, but the practice had ceased in the aftermath of that earlier conflict.[116] The Americans had continued to use nurse-anaesthetists in the inter-war period and, according to Parsons, there were a number of British medical officers who, having worked with these nurses, were impressed by the service that they were able to provide.[117] This did not assuage the anger of several correspondents to the *British Medical Journal.* A.M. Barford's letter, published on 5 October 1940, stated that 'the employment for this can be no other than a retrograde step … I hope I shall never be a patient there, and I venture to say that each one of them [medical staff] would not wish a nurse to give him an anaesthetic.'[118] W. Stanley-Sykes wrote of nurse-anaesthetists as being the 'bane of the second-rate American medical school' and praised the Canadians for outlawing the practice.[119] Despite such antagonism to the idea of nurse-anaesthetists, there was a caveat to the correspondence from one medical man, that although nurses should not replace medically trained anaesthetists, they could perhaps give anaesthetics for 'minor surgical work'.[120] What constituted 'minor' or major surgery on active service overseas was meaningless. Army nurses shifted the boundaries of their surgical practice as the exigencies of war demanded, and neither they nor their medical colleagues showed any of the professional anxieties of their counterparts on home soil.

After being shipwrecked on the *SS Kuala*, following the escape from Singapore in February 1942, Sister Edith Stevenson and her fellow passengers, found themselves island-hopping to avoid detection by the Japanese:

> We knew those who had infected wounds would die and there was one case of gangrene needing amputation ... One other nurse and myself had been trained in operating theatre work, we knew the procedures but we had neither the instruments or anaesthetic.
>
> One morning as if in answer to a prayer, a doctor Kirkwood arrived. What a relief to see him and his two orderlies. They had left Singapore after the Japanese invasion, travelling in a small motor-boat, they flew the Red Cross Flag and the Japanese allowed them safe passage. The doctor decided to amputate the leg as soon as we could make preparations. He had ether and chloroform and a few instruments. Strangely enough, he had no scissors, I was glad I had mine. We had no steriliser, so I found an empty kerosene tin and boiled the instruments in this over a charcoal brasier [*sic*], it was all very unorthodox. Doctor had some dressings and when all was ready we began. We were in the open air. Doctor started the anaesthetic and then handed over to his orderly whilst he began the operation. We amputated the leg and were just about ready to stitch up the flap of skin round the stump when the orderly flopped to the ground in a faint. The smell of the anaesthetic, together with an empty stomach proved too much for him. I took over the anaesthetic and doctor finished the stitching. The second orderly attended to his colleague.[121]

Following the capture of the ship the *Rangitane*, a group of nursing sisters were amongst the only British military women during the whole war[122] to be held in captivity by Germans. The German sailors appear to have been profoundly uncomfortable holding them as prisoners. Whilst the men were taken below deck, the nurses were placed in a 'wooden structure on deck'. The German sailors had been preparing to lock the door, but an appeal by the nurses not to do so was accepted and 'we were left with guards after a drink of good hot coffee with sugar and milk'.[123] The nurses, aware of the levels of illness and injury on board, sent to the German ship's doctor to ask if they could help:

> Very quickly we were in his surgery … The doctor gave the anaesthetics and then left Sister to keep the patient under, carefully explaining that nurses did not do that work in Germany. 'Nor in England' we answered him. When we got there he was just finishing inspecting the wounds, and, with our help was able to begin operating on the serious cases at once.[124]

Evelyn Cottrell, a nursing sister with the Spears Unit,[125] was part of the contingent of nurses at the battle of Monte Cassino:

> That was a very gruesome time, we had so many casualties, errm, so many casualties brought to us that they were all laid out the length of this room in rows and the colonel and the other doctors went round and the ones they thought they could save, they worked on, and the ones they, they couldn't do anything for, they hadn't time to do anything for and we used to dig out bits of shrapnel and err errm give blood all the time, we were always giving blood transfusions and err salines and things like that and we did a lot of minor surgery really with err, well with shrapnel bits and things and we didn't sleep, we just worked day and night and the colonel operated and operated day and night and had sort of an hour's sleep and off again and they were working like mad and a lot of people died, but a lot of people he saved, that wouldn't have been saved if they'd had to go back any further.[126]

These three separate and quite different accounts are critical for demonstrating the very different attitudes of doctors and nurses on active service to their perhaps more conservative colleagues in Britain. First, the admission by Stevenson that, had she had instruments and a means of anaesthesia, she and her nurse colleague would have operated on the severely injured man themselves suggests a willingness to ignore professionally held beliefs about what constituted nursing or medical work. Second, none of the incidents created any anxieties between either the medical practitioners or the nursing staff; all seemingly worked to the conviction that professional boundaries should not be maintained for the sake of the injured patients. Third, it was the male orderly who fainted, not the female nurse. Although the multiple gender contradictions that arose in the Second World War remained a source of concern for those keen to preserve the status quo, episodes like these identify the vital importance that such inter-professional concerns were ignored and, perhaps more pertinently, that they were no longer deemed appropriate. On active service overseas, British nursing sisters and their medical colleagues clearly believed it was the nurses' duty to expand their roles, despite professional and gendered notions, and that the most important person in the equation was the patient, not the nurse and not the doctor.

Thus far in this chapter the focus has been on duties that extended the province of nurses' work, such as their increasing responsibility for complex wounds, and on work that was an expansion of the nursing role into what had been previously considered medical work, for example, blood transfusions and the participation of nursing staff in anaesthetics. There was, however, one area of practice that would necessitate collaborative working, that required both professions to learn together almost from the beginning, and that did not enter the lexicon of medical work until 1942 – penicillin.

New work: 'The new wonder drug Penicillin'

Penicillin was made available to military patients in 1943 and was arguably the 'most significant achievement of the Second World War science and technology'.[127] It was also a critical intervention for nurses, despite some initial fears. Prior to its development, often the only way to save a patient's life was through careful, meticulous and time-consuming nursing. Once penicillin became available it was as if nursing had 'gone out of the window'.[128] Since their discovery and production in 1935, the sulphonamide drugs that were the precursors to penicillin had proved highly useful chemotherapeutic agents for the inhibition of certain bacteria. Sulphanilamide was effective against streptococcal infections, sulphapyridine against pneumococcal infections, gonorrhoea and meningitis, and sulphaguanidine successfully treated some cases of dysentery.[129]

However, a number of problems with the sulphonamides meant that they were not the ideal drug therapies. For many patients they led to nausea and vomiting, and for others, depression, dizziness and headaches were also common. By 1943 a paper appeared in the medical press alerting doctors to the possibility of allergic reactions to the sulpha drugs.[130] More serious, but not as common, were the side-effects of agranulocytosis and haemolytic anaemia. In the former, reduced white cell counts were noted that led to ulceration of the mouth and throat and a general deterioration in the patient's condition. The latter manifested as jaundice and haemoglobinuria.[131] According to C.M. Fletcher of the Radcliffe Infirmary at Oxford, whilst the sulpha drugs had 'revolutionized many parts of medicine', their potentially 'severely poisonous effects' meant that 'no one could claim that they were ideal'.[132] Importantly, penicillin could cure staphylococcus infections which the sulpha drugs could not. Furthermore, its safety was believed in absolutely,[133] and any early problems were blamed on the production process rather than on the drug itself.[134] It was not until 1945 that a paper appeared in the *British Medical Journal* informing readers of the possibility of allergic reactions, warning that 'it is understood that the above is the only occurrence of a reaction of this type [eczema and discharge] to penicillin therapy in more than 30,000 cases treated in the B.L.A. [British Liberation Army]'.[135] Despite such ardent confidence in the marvel of penicillin, in its very early days there were some substantial problems. Florey and his team struggled to produce it in sufficient quantities. Moreover, penicillin was so rapidly excreted by the kidneys that in the very early experimental uses on patients in England, staff had to collect the patient's urine and extract the penicillin to provide further doses.[136] From these very early experiments, it was realised that the co-operation and interest of the nursing staff was essential.[137]

Although penicillin was available from 1943, as one report in the *British Journal of Nursing* maintained, 'its manufacture even in minute quantities is so tedious and lengthy that the entire output is reserved for the Services'.[138] One effect of this, which caused consternation in the press and amongst practitioners in the field, was that its use for the military meant that it was available for German POWs[139] but not British civilians, even those whose injuries were war related. According to a brief report in the *British Medical Journal*, 'the Government was required by the Geneva Convention to care for wounded prisoners of war, without distinction of nationality, equally with our own personnel', and there was just not enough available to treat both the military and civilians.[140] Despite this pronouncement, there were occasional experiments with penicillin on members of the civilian population, although it was used only as a '"corpse-raising drug," i.e., not being tried until all else has failed'.[141]

In December 1943, *The Lancet* reported that Florey and his team had been in North Africa since the summer, testing the efficacy of penicillin. They demonstrated that it was effective on all soft-tissue wounds, including septic wounds, and that a combatant infected with gonorrhoea could be treated and returned to the front within three days.[142] By 1944, it was more generally used in war zones, but not without its difficulties for both the nursing staff and the patients themselves. According to much of the analysis in the nursing and medical press, it could not be given orally and its rapid excretion meant that it needed to be given as intramuscular injections at three-hourly intervals.[143] The injections were very painful, repetitive and interrupted the combatant patient's much-needed sleep.[144] Alternatively it could be given as a constant intravenous infusion,[145] but this required very careful nursing attention and a medical presence to site the infusion cannula, both of which could be difficult on active service overseas. In February 1945, Sister M.K.I. Harpin wrote to Dame Katharine Jones maintaining that a method of administering penicillin orally to a patient with pneumonia had been used and had worked, although it still required a three-hourly intervention and could not have been pleasant for the patient:

> A level teaspoonful of alkali – which in this case was magnesium trisilicate or sodium bicarbonate, was taken dissolved in a quarter of a pint of milk. Ten minutes later the Penicillin beaten up with an egg, and with a little milk and glucose added was given. This procedure was repeated three hourly, each dose being followed by a mouth wash.[146]

For those nurses and doctors seeing penicillin in use in the early days, it was like a miracle. Morris described it as 'The new wonder drug Penicillin', which, she wrote, was 'a great help in the fight to save the lives of young men like Len. This is the first time I have seen the antibiotic in action … It seems particularly good in preventing gangrene infections in gunshot wounds.'[147] However, in October 1944 Morris had another patient whose infected stump did not appear to respond to penicillin.[148] Unfortunately she does not follow up this case in her diary, so it is not known whether the treatment was eventually successful or not. Bolton's war memoir records the first time she saw penicillin used, sometime in the spring of 1944, whilst nursing in India:

> Major Niblock and Joan Inman were there, dressed as for an operation in gauze masks, sterile gowns and rubber gloves. The major was drawing some yellow liquid into a large syringe. He held it up to the light, saying, 'This is the new drug, which has just arrived. It is called Penicillin and we are going to try it on this patient.' After carefully cleaning the skin, he injected the drug into a muscle ... Just before going off duty we visited the ward once more and were astonished at the improved state of the wound. There was no longer any doubt – the infection was receding. After five days of three-hourly injections the solider was able to walk with the help of a stick, finally making a complete recovery.[149]

Bolton does not say who administered the three-hourly injections to this man, but it is unlikely that it was the doctor. Other nurses across all the war zones of the globe described the arduous and time-consuming nature of penicillin administration. Gertrude Cooper, a Queen Alexandra's Royal Naval Nursing Service Sister, described the work entailed in administering it intramuscularly: 'the penicillin was um, solid – it floats sufficiently to draw it up into a syringe already loaded with um – saline, and when this mixture was mixed it was given in the buttock'.[150] According to Dyer, 'it had to be given three hourly day and night which meant a constant flow of work preparing, sterilising, and giving injections and no sooner had we completed one round of injections to the various patients when it was time to start the next'.[151] Salter's testimony corroborates the elaborate and time-consuming work, administered as it was 'at three hourly intervals under full aseptic conditions'.[152] Even when the orders for strict asepsis were abandoned, the need for the drug to be given three hourly meant that the work remained time consuming. It would not have been possible, therefore, for the medical officers to continue to be the professionals who administered it. Nevertheless, their continued interest in its usage and the rapid involvement of the nursing staff in its administration suggest growing acknowledgement of the professional abilities and trustworthiness of nursing sisters.[153] Critically, penicillin if administered early in the infection, whether that infection was caused by illness or injury, could return men very rapidly to war.[154] The need for nurses to administer penicillin thus legitimated their place in volatile, front-line duty. Nursing sisters were therefore able to 'parlay' their skills with this new technology to be included in forward areas.

The whole ethos of penicillin in the Second World War seems to have been one of inter-professional participation.[155] PMRAFNS Sister Joan Peake recalled that the chemists in the pharmacy at her Cairo hospital made 'primitive penicillin by growing a mould on jam, pots of jam, used to sterilise it and send it up to use and we used to use it on desert sores, with exceptionally good results'.[156] By December 1943, the *British Medical Journal* was detailing that such practices were not supported: 'the Mediterranean Report urges strict control of supplies, with concentration in one theatre of operations, and gives no encouragement to the supporters of crude penicillin'.[157] According to Cynthia Toman, having learnt about penicillin on active service overseas alongside their medical colleagues, Canadian nursing sisters returned to civilian practice in the post-war era and there played an important role in teaching medical staff about the drug.[158] Such activity altered both gender and professional boundaries in a way that would have not been considered possible prior to the Second World War. There is no evidence in the personal testimonies of British nurses that this was mirrored in Britain. However, it is likely, given the close involvement of nursing sisters in all war zones in the preparation, administration and monitoring of penicillin, that they were called upon to train nurses and doctors who had not been on active service overseas in its use.

Conclusion

The constantly shifting requirements of war nursing prevented Army nurses from remaining in a professional comfort zone of accepted roles and regimes. The experience of living with uncertainty may have caused anxieties for some, but the active participation in new treatment modalities suggests that nurses who went to war were keen to move beyond the normal boundaries of nursing practice and many relished the opportunity to do so. The chapter has examined a range of surgical practices by way of a 'case study' of changing nursing roles. Whether they arose from traditional nursing work that was altered by the exigencies of war, were work that the over-stretched but now trusting medical staff passed on to nursing sisters or were roles that by reason of their novelty were developed by the medical and nursing staff as a team, the new responsibilities raised the nurses' sense of their professional ability.

Despite the increased confidence and autonomy in practice, the war was not the watershed for nursing that some have argued.[159] Some of the extended, expanded and new work was, by the end of the war, enshrined into nursing practice; other work was reclaimed by and returned to medicine. The differentiations of these working practices, and the reasons why some were given gladly to the nurses, such as blood transfusion work, while other work was closely re-guarded at the end of the war by medics, have been the subject of a number of texts.[160] What was critical to the professional lives of British Army nurses who were posted overseas during the Second World War was that, despite the challenges inherent in the negotiations of work and gender boundaries, they were changed by them. For many, in the aftermath of war, a return to the stifled world of the British hospital nursing system was not possible, and many sought alternatives.

Notes

1 Brenda McBryde, *A Nurse's War* (Saffron Walden: Cakebread Publications, 1993), 57.
2 Joan E. Lynaugh and Julie Fairman, *Critical Care Nursing: A History* (Philadelphia, PA: University of Pennsylvania Press, 1998), 11.
3 Lucy Noakes, *War and the British: Gender, Memory and National Identity* (London: I.B. Tauris, 1998), 52.
4 Noakes, *War and the British*, 20–1.
5 War Office, 'No. 1 General Hospital Jan to December 1940' (23 April 1940), TNA WO 177/1092.
6 Cynthia Toman, *An Officer and a Lady: Canadian Military Nursing and the Second World War* (Vancouver: University of British Columbia Press, 2007), 57.
7 Cynthia Toman, 'Front lines and frontiers: War as legitimate work for nurses, 1939–1945', *Social History* 40, 79 (2007): 72.
8 Anonymous Sister (QAIMNS/R), 'The departure of the British Military Hospital, Marseilles', in Ada Harrison (ed.), *Grey and Scarlet: Letters from the War Areas by Army Sisters on Active Service* (London: Hodder and Stoughton, 1944), 21.
9 Mary Morris, 'The diary of a wartime nurse' (23 June 1944), 107, IWM

Documents 4850; Mary Morris, *A Very Private Diary: A Nurse in Wartime*, ed. Carol Acton (London: Weidenfeld and Nicolson, 2014), 93.

10 Sister TANS, 'Experiences of an Army Sister in the Middle East', MMM QARANC uncatalogued archive, MEF memoirs.

11 Betty C. Parkin, *Desert Nurse: A World War II Memoir* (London: Robert Hale, 1990), 131.

12 Angela Bolton, *The Maturing Sun: An Army Nurse in India 1942–45* (London: Headline, 1986), 195.

13 Anonymous Sister, 'Middle East and the hospital at Tobruk', in Ada Harrison (ed.), *Grey and Scarlet: Letters From the War Areas by Army Sisters on Active Service* (London: Hodder and Stoughton, 1944), 126; Geraldine Edge and Mary E. Johnston, *Ships of Youth: The Experiences of Two Army Nursing Sisters on Board the Hospital Carrier Leinster* (London: Hodder and Stoughton, 1945), 45.

14 Morris, 'The diary of a wartime nurse' (20 February 1945).

15 Esther Helen Audrey Luker ARRC, 'Diaries from 1940–45' (7 November 1940), IWM Documents 1274.

16 Luker 'Diaries' (20 December 1940)

17 Parkin, *Desert Nurse*, 115.

18 Catherine Arnold Hutchinson, 'My war and welcome to it', 112, IWM Documents 11950.

19 Joan Eileen Nicolson, oral history by Conrad Wood, 8 June 1991, IWM Sound Archive 12075.

20 Ana Carden-Coyne, *The Politics of Wounds: Military Patients and Medical Power in the First World War* (Oxford: Oxford University Press, 2014), 301–2.

21 According to Anna Rogers, the New Zealand orderlies were initially highly circumspect about working under the authority of nursing sisters, having never worked under a woman before. However, Rogers argues, the orderlies were ultimately glad of the nursing sisters' expert knowledge of nursing matters to guide them. Anna Rogers, *While You're Away: New Zealand Nurses at War, 1899–1948* (Auckland: Auckland University Press, 2003), 212. It is likely that this change in attitude was not quite as stark as Rogers maintains, and that there remained many male orderlies for whom the advent of nursing sisters into their masculine domain was an affront. However, the posting of nursing sisters to forward areas, including Mobile Dressing Stations, suggests that the benefit of expert female nurses outweighed any personal feelings. Rogers, *While You're Away*, 239.

22 Emma Newlands, *Civilians into Soldiers: War, the Body and British Army Recruits, 1939–45* (Manchester: Manchester University Press, 2014), 131.

23 Toman, *An Officer and a Lady*, 118; Kevin Brown, *Fighting Fit: Health, Medicine and War in the Twentieth Century* (Stroud: The History Press, 2008, Kindle edition), loc. 3099.

24 Julie Fairman and Patricia D'Antonio, 'Reimagining nursing's place in the history of clinical practice', *Journal of the History of Medicine and Allied Health Sciences* 63, 4 (2008): 444.
25 Toman, *An Officer and a Lady*, 64.
26 Margarete Sandelowski, 'Venous envy: The post-World War II debate over IV nursing', *Advances in Nursing Science* 22, 1 (1999): 52–62; Margarete Sandelowski, *Devices and Desires: Gender, Technology and American Nursing* (Chapel Hill, NC: University of North Carolina Press, 2000).
27 Apart from the tasks discussed in this chapter, other key therapies that became part of the nurses' lexicon of skills on active service overseas were monitoring of the effects of new psychotherapeutic treatment regimes and the microscopic diagnosis of malaria. For a detailed discussion of the war work of Hildegard Peplau, the pioneering mental health nurse, with psychologically damaged men, see especially, Barbara J. Callaway, *Hildegard Peplau: Psychiatric Nurse of the Century* (New York: Springer, 2002). Patricia Moody described the interest she gained from learning to read malaria slides: 'I am learning bacteriology and spend a fair amount of my spare time peering down a microscope searching blood slides looking for malarial parasites.' Sister Patricia Moody TANS, 'My dearest mums', 76 General Hospital, British North Africa Force (24 July 1943) RCN Archives, Edinburgh. Tropical disease diagnosis and treatment had become the province of the nurses, who appear to have taken to the new role with willingness. This work was time consuming, required precision in the timing of taking blood slides and placed the responsibility for reading the results of the slide with the nurses themselves. Toman, *An Officer and a Lady*, 134.
28 According to Ana Carden-Coyne, 'Blighty' was first used to describe Britain as home in the First World War. It originated in colonial India, 'belati' being the Hindustani word for 'home; foreign country'. The British then punned with 'blight'. Carden-Coyne, *The Politics of Wounds*, 71.
29 David Justham, '"Those maggots – they did a wonderful job": The nurses' role in wound management in civilian hospitals during the Second World War', in Jane Brooks and Christine E. Hallett (eds), *One Hundred Years of Nursing Wartime Practices, 1854–1953* (Manchester: Manchester University Press, 2015), 198. Testimonies from nursing sisters maintained that this disciplined training had supported the sublimation of the self into a 'nursing-self', thus enabling them to undertake dirty work and also work under the intense pressure needed for war nursing. For a detailed discussion of the benefits of the dehumanising and disciplined training of nurses, see Chapter 1 in this volume.
30 Michael Traynor, Maggie Boland and Niels Buus, 'Autonomy, evidence and intuition: Nurses and decision-making', *Journal of Advanced Nursing* 66, 7 (2010): 1584–91.
31 Justham, '"Those maggots – they did a wonderful job"', 194. Although

some nurses would not alter the round, depending on which wounds were clean or dirty, there were other hospitals in which they were expected to make such decisions. Justham, '"Those maggots – they did a wonderful job"', 193.

32 Morris, 'The diary of a wartime nurse' (31 May 1940), 2; Morris, *A Very Private Diary*, 3.

33 Penny Salter, 'Long ago and far away: A distant memory': A diary, c. 1938–1970, 24–6, UK Centre for the History of Nursing (UKCHN), University of Manchester. See also IWM Documents 17649.

34 Mary Bond, *Wartime Experiences from the Midnight Sun to Belsen* (Cardigan: E.L. Jones and Son, 1994), 16.

35 Toman argues that this conveyor-belt 'care' that was a part of wartime nursing, exemplified 'dirty' work. It was mundane, physically dirty and repetitious. This understanding of body work which renders it low status and designated as women's work is developed in Jocalyn Lawler's *Behind the Screens: Nursing, Somology and the Problem of the Body* (Melbourne: Churchill Livingstone, 1991) and discussed with reference to nursing wartime work by Jane Brooks and Christine E. Hallett, 'Introduction: The practice of nursing and the exigencies of war', in Jane Brooks and Christine E. Hallett (eds), *One Hundred Years of Wartime Nursing Practices, 1854–1953* (Manchester: Manchester University Press, 2015). However, there is no suggestion in any of the testimonies that the British nurses in the Second World War understood it that way, especially when left to the work without interference from authority. In fact, when Sister Agnes Morgan is left to face a convoy at her CCS in Europe, she described the excitement of working under 'real war-nursing' conditions and how they just 'got down to our endless stream of wounded men'. Agnes Kathleen Dunbar Morgan, 'My dearest mums', letter 57 (August 1943), CMF, 2. 'Still with the lamp: letters to my mother by an army nursing sister. Egypt – North Africa – Sicily – Italy, 1941–1944', IWM Documents 16686. As Julie Anderson acknowledges, improved transport technologies meant that men could access more complex treatment in mobile units. The increasing complexity of the treatments in turn meant that registered nurses were needed to care for the men, moving the nursing sisters ever closer to the battle lines. Julie Anderson, *War, Disability and Rehabilitation in Britain: 'Soul of a Nation'* (Manchester: Manchester University Press, 2011), 76.

36 J.R. Learmonth, 'The surgical nurse', in J.M. Mackintosh (ed.), *Wartime Nurse: An Anthology of Ideas about the Care and Nursing of War Casualties* (Edinburgh: Oliver and Boyd, 1940), 22.

37 Bruce M. Dick, 'Injuries and wounds of the chest', in J.M. Mackintosh (ed.), *Wartime Nurse: An Anthology of Ideas about the Care and Nursing of War Casualties* (Edinburgh: Oliver and Boyd, 1940), 85.

38 John Elam, 'Anaesthesia in war-time', *The Lancet* (15 April 1939): 906.

39 Morris, 'The diary of a wartime nurse' (7 September 1944), 130; Morris, *A Very Private Diary*, 112.
40 Carden-Coyne, *The Politics of Wounds*,191.
41 E.L. L'Estrainge, 'Work and experiences in the Middle East, 1941–1942', MMM QARANC uncatalogued archive, MEF memoirs.
42 W.H.C. Romanis, 'Amputation in war time', *Nursing Times* (15 June 1940): 266.
43 Sister TANS, 'Experiences of an Army Sister in the Middle East'.
44 H.B. Woods, 'Treatment of severe war-time burns', *Nursing Times* (5 November 1943): 833.
45 Morris, 'The diary of a wartime nurse' (5 October 1944), 144; Morris, *A Very Private Diary*, 126–7.
46 T.B. Layton, 'Transport of wounded: Surgical aspects', *The Lancet* (23 March 1940): 537–40.
47 Hutchinson, 'My war and welcome to it', 40.
48 Dorothy B. Doughty, 'History of ostomy surgery', *Journal of Wound Ostomy Continence Nursing* 35, 1 (2008): 34–8.
49 *The Feminine Touch*. Director, Pat Jackson, written by Iain MacCormick. Released 27 March 1956, Ealing Studios. The film follows the lives of five student nurses in the young NHS. http://www.imdb.com/title/tt0050428/ [accessed 28 September 2016].
50 Julia Hallam identifies this film as one in which the nurse's role as patient carer is subordinated to nurse as the one who cares for the male doctor, thereby playing into post-war tropes of a domesticity. Nevertheless, as Hallam argues, 'the deep happiness to be found in nursing is that of being in service'. Julia Hallam, *Nursing the Image: Media, Culture and Professional Identity* (London: Routledge, 2000), 61.
51 Hutchinson, 'My war and welcome to it', 39.
52 McBryde, *A Nurse's War*, 58.
53 Sister N.M. Liddiard, 'Surgical nursing in wartime' (3 September 1945), MMM QARANC uncatalogued archive.
54 Cecil P.G. Wakeley, 'The treatment of war burns', *Nursing Times* (11 December 1941): 819.
55 R.G. Henderson, 'Treatment of incendiary bomb burns', *Nursing Mirror* (6 July 1940): 325.
56 Anonymous, 'Editorial: Tannic acid "is out"', *Nursing Mirror and Midwives Journal* (23 November 1940):171. For a detailed discussion of the debates about the use of tannic acid in the early 1940s, see Brown, *Fighting Fit*, loc. 2318–3244.
57 Anonymous, 'Editorial: Tannic acid "is out"', 171. According to Mayhew, it was McIndoe himself who secured the banning of tannic acid. Emily Mayhew, *The Reconstruction of Warriors: Archibald McIndoe, The Royal Air Force and the Guinea Pig Club* (Barnsley: Greenhill Books, 2010, Kindle edition), loc.

900–921. Harrison maintains that a study by the Medical Research Council that highlighted the liver damage that it caused ultimately led to its demise. Mark Harrison, *Medicine and Victory: British Military Medicine in the Second World War* (Oxford: Oxford University Press, 2004), 157.

58 Morris, 'The diary of a wartime nurse' (1 June 1940), 2; Morris, *A Very Private Diary*, 4.

59 John Bunyan, 'A preliminary report on treatment of wounds and burns by the envelope method', *Nursing Mirror* 72 (22 February 1941): supplement, ii–iii.

60 Anonymous Nursing Sister, 'The adventures of a nursing officer (QAIMNS) 1939–45 and sidelights of some tropical diseases, also battle wounds', MMM QARANC uncatalogued archive, MEF memoirs.

61 Anonymous QAIMNS Reserve, 'Gibraltar, January 1940 to January 1942', in Ada Harrison (ed.), *Grey and Scarlet: Letters from the War Areas by Army Sisters on Active Service* (London: Hodder and Stoughton, 1944), 136–7.

62 V. Shennan, 'Notes on the treatment of burns with sulphonamide "emulsion" in a base hospital M.E.F.', MMM QARANC uncatalogued archive.

63 Stanford Cade, 'Burns in the Royal Air Force', *Medical Training Establishment and Dept Royal Air Force Journal* 1 (1941): 2.

64 Emergency Medical Services, Ministry of Health, 'Memorandum: The treatment of burns', *Nursing Times* (5 April 1941): 242.

65 Penny Starns, *Nurses at War: Women on the Frontline, 1939–45* (Stroud: Sutton Publishing, 2000), 41.

66 Archibald H. McIndoe, 'Saline baths treatment for burns', *Nursing Mirror* (18 July 1942): i.

67 McIndoe, 'Saline baths treatment for burns', ii.

68 Bolton, *The Maturing Sun*, 168.

69 Ann Radloff, 'Going to Gooseberry Beach: Travels and adventures of a nursing sister', 5, IWM 147.

70 Betty Evans oral history interview by Jane Brooks via the telephone on 10 January 2014.

71 Edge and Johnston, *Ships of Youth*, 118.

72 Norman J. Logie, 'Treatment of burns at Tobruk', *The Lancet* (15 May 1943): 609.

73 Logie, 'Treatment of burns at Tobruk', 611.

74 Evans, oral history, 10 January 2014.

75 Philip Mitchiner, 'Modern methods of treating war burns', *Nursing Mirror* (10 May 1943): 23.

76 Woods, 'Treatment of severe war-time burns', 821.

77 Woods, 'Treatment of severe war-time burns', 827.

78 Evans, oral history, 10 January 2014.

79 Anonymous Nursing Sister, 'The Anzio Beachhead', MMM QARANC uncatalogued archive, CMF file.

80 Anonymous, 'The technique of blood transfusion', *Nursing Mirror* (2 September 1939): 764.

81 P.M. Dyer, 'When life was grey and scarlet: A recollection of life as an Army Nursing Sister', 71, MMM QARANC/PE/1/151/DYER Box 8.

82 June Hamilton, oral history interview by Jane Brooks at her home in the South of England, 19 October 2011.

83 Sandelowski, 'Venous envy', 57.

84 McBryde, *A Nurse's War*, 86.

85 Toman, *An Officer and a Lady*, 126.

86 Harold Smith's assertion that Arthur Marwick was mistaken when he assumed that the war altered the position of women is in many ways borne out in the reality that women in healthcare were maintained in nursing rather than encouraged to enter the medical profession. However, Smith's notion that this lack of opportunity did not manifest itself in an altered consciousness of women is more difficult to substantiate. Women may have continued to be nurses next to the undoubtedly academically, financially and socially superior medical profession, but the war certainly altered the way they understood themselves in the medical team. Harold Smith, 'The effect of the war on the status of women', in Harold Smith (ed.), *War and Social Change: British Society in the Second World War* (Manchester: Manchester University Press, 1986), 217.

87 Agnes Morgan's brother was a medical doctor, P.M. Dyer's brother was an officer in the RAF.

88 Mary Morris wrote humorously and without deference of the arrival of a gynaecologist as the new medical officer to their hospital in August 1944: 'there is bound to be a certain amount of culture shock for him here!' Morris, 'The diary of a wartime nurse' (31 August 1944), 128. Such statements leave the reader with the genuine impression that those already experienced in battle conditions believed themselves to be superior in knowledge to newly posted colleagues, whatever their professional background. See also Morris, *A Very Private Diary*, 110. Cynthia Toman argues that the Canadian nurses experienced a similar rise in confidence as they were trusted to take on increasingly experimental, innovative and complex work. Toman, 'Front lines and frontiers', 66.

89 Geraldine Edge and Mary Johnston note that when they landed in Italy in 1943, 'the anaesthetist and surgeon would go to the wards and give plasma or a blood transfusion'. Edge and Johnston, *Ships of Youth*, 33.

90 Carden-Coyne, *The Politics of Wounds*, 146; Christine E. Hallett, *Containing Trauma: Nursing Work in the First World War* (Manchester: Manchester University Press, 2009), 31–2. Hallett describes the two most popular techniques, firstly the one favoured by Canadian physician Lawrence Bruce Robertson, in which the doctor withdrew blood from the donor in a canula and then injected into the recipient via another canula. The other technique

involved blood being allowed to flow freely directly from the donor into the recipient.

91 Carden-Coyne, *The Politics of Wounds*, 147; Hallett, *Containing Trauma*, 32.

92 Carden-Coyne, *The Politics of Wounds*, 156.

93 Ian Whitehead, 'The British medical officer on the Western Front', in Roger Cooter, Mark Harrison and Steve Sturdy (eds), *Medicine and Modern Warfare* (Amsterdam, Atlanta: Rodopi, 1999), 171.

94 Angela Jackson, 'Blood and guts: Nursing with the International Brigades in the Spanish Civil War, 1936–39', in Jane Brooks and Christine E. Hallett (eds), *One Hundred Years of Nursing Wartime Practices, 1854–1953* (Manchester: Manchester University Press, 2015), 172.

95 Cynthia Toman, 'Blood work: Canadian nursing and blood transfusion, 1942–1990', *Nursing History Review* 9 (2001): 52.

96 Margaret R. Higonnet and Patrice L.-R. Higonnet, 'The double helix', in Margaret Randolph Higonnet, Jane Jenson, Sonya Michel and Margaret Collins Weitz (eds), *Behind the Lines: Gender and the Two World Wars* (New Haven, CT: Yale University Press, 1987).

97 Penny Summerfield, 'Gender and war in the twentieth century', *The International History Review* 19, 1 (1997): 4.

98 D.M. Long, 'Advances in surgical nursing, with special reference to work in C.C.S. etc.', 1, MMM QARACNC uncatalogued archive.

99 Toman, *An Officer and a Lady*, 143.

100 Julie Fairman, 'Alterative visions: the nurse–technology relationship in the context of the history of technology', *Nursing History Review* 6 (1998): 137.

101 Mark Harrison, *Medicine and Victory: British Military Medicine in the Second World War* (Oxford: Oxford University Press, 2004), 116. Contrary to this belief, however, it is apparent that in some circumstances plasma continued to be used for shock, instead of blood. On 23 June 1944, Mary Morris wrote in her diary, 'The ones who were shocked through loss of blood were put on a plasma intravenous drip'. Morris, 'The diary of a wartime nurse' (23 June 1944), 108; Morris, *A Very Private Diary*, 93.

102 F.A.E. Crew, '25. The Field Transfusion Unit: United Kingdom – the Army', in Arthur Salusbury MacNalty and W. Franklin Mellor (eds), *Medical Services in War: The Principal Medical Lessons of the Second World War* (London: HMSO, 1968), 123.

103 Emily Soper, oral history interview via telephone by Jane Brooks, 6 September 2013.

104 Harrison, *Medicine and Victory*, 56; Brown, *Fighting Fit*, loc. 3262.

105 C.A. Wells, 'Post-war pattern: War-time advances in surgery', *Nursing Times* (9 June 1945): 369.

106 Anonymous, 'Editorial: War-time advances and antiseptics', *Nursing Times* (11 April 1942): 237.

107 Morris, 'The diary of a wartime nurse' (4 October 1944), 143; Morris (Acton ed.), *A Very Private Diary*, 125.
108 Harrison, *Medicine and Victory*, 115.
109 Anonymous Nursing Sister, 'The adventures of a nursing officer', 14.
110 L'Estrainge, 'Work and experiences in the Middle East, 1941–1942'.
111 Anonymous, 'In step with the QAs. 8. - Hospital ship (Part I), *Nursing Times* (30 September 1944): 678. For a more detailed discussion of the involvement of orderlies in blood transfusion work see 'David Proctor, RAMC, orderly, 1944–47', in Barbara Mortimer, *Sisters: Extraordinary True-Life Stories from Nurses in World War Two* (London: Hutchinson, 2012), 198–9. In 1947, David Proctor entered St Mary's Hospital, Highgate, London to train as a State Registered Nurse. Whilst it was still unusual for men to enter general nursing at this time, men were coming out of the forces wanting to train as nurses and therefore a small but significant body of men in general nursing began to emerge. Mortimer, *Sisters*, 299.
112 Toman, 'Blood work'.
113 Nurse anaesthetists had been trained the First World War by Britain, the Dominions and the USA. Although, because of the antipathy of the Australian Director of Medical Services towards women being posted to forward areas, Australian nurses were never allowed to actually practise, all the other nations used nurses to provide ether anaesthetics. At the end of the war, only the USA continued to use nurses in this role. Hallett, *Containing Trauma*, 99–100; Carden-Coyne, *The Politics of Wounds*, 76.
114 F.B. Parsons, 'Nurse anaesthetists', *British Medical Journal* (28 September 1940): 429.
115 Parsons, 'Nurse anaesthetists', 429.
116 Hallett, *Containing Trauma*, 99.
117 Parsons, 'Nurse anaesthetists', 429.
118 A.M. Barford, 'Nurse anaesthetics', *British Medical Journal* (5 October 1940): 474.
119 W. Stanley-Sykes, 'Nurse anaesthetists', *British Medical Journal* (1 March 1941): 339.
120 Alan F. Goode, 'Correspondence', *British Medical Journal* (28 September 1940): 430.
121 Edith Stevenson, 'The last lap: Autobiography 1912–1986', 14–15. IWM LBY94/1636.
122 Whilst there may have been other incidences, this was the only one found during the research for this book.
123 Anonymous, 'Nursing adventure: The story of two nursing sisters returning on the Torpedoed "*Rangitane*"', *Nursing Times* (25 October 1942): 672.
124 Anonymous, 'Nursing adventure', 672.
125 The Spears Unit was accredited to the Free French Forces and under the

command of Lady Spears, formerly Mary Borden, and Lady Hadfield. See Eric Taylor, *Front-Line Nurse: British Nurses in World War II* (London, Robert Hale, 1997), 39; Christine E. Hallett, *Nurse Writers of the Great War* (Manchester: Manchester University Press, 2016), 58.

126 Evelyn Alma Cottrell, Spears Unit, oral history interview by Lyn E. Smith, 9 July 1990, IWM Oral History Collection, Interview 12180.

127 Peter Neushul, 'Fighting research: Army participation in the clinical testing and mass production of penicillin during the Second World War', in Roger Cooter, Mark Harrison and Steve Sturdy (eds), *War, Medicine and Modernity* (Stroud: Sutton Publishing, 1998), 204. See also Harrison, *Medicine and Victory*; Mayhew, *The Reconstruction of Warriors*, loc. 436; Brown, *Fighting Fit*.

128 Winifred Hector, in Barbara Mortimer, *Sisters: Extraordinary True-Life Stories from Nurses in World War Two* (London: Hutchinson, 2012), 196. The notion that penicillin would reduce the need for nurses and might even put the profession in peril is also discussed in Starns, *Nurses at War*, in which Monica Baly is cited as stating, 'No longer was the doctor saying, "I can't do anything, but nursing will do a great deal". We had now got to the stage when it appeared as if nursing was not doing very much. The patients got better whether they were nursed or not.' Starns, *Nurses at War*, 72. See also Justham, '"Those maggots – they did a wonderful job"'.

129 John F. Stokes, 'The present status of the sulphonamide drugs', *Nursing Times* (21 February 1942): 124; S.C. Turner, 'All in the day's work. III – Nursing on a troopship', *Nursing Times* (17 January 1942): 76.

130 R.G. Park, 'Cutaneous hypersensitivity to sulphonamides: A report of 12 cases', *The British Medical Journal* 2, 4306 (17 July 1943): 69–72.

131 Stokes, 'The present status of the sulphonamide drugs', 125.

132 C.M. Fletcher, 'Penicillin: A recent advance in chemotherapy', *Nursing Times* (4 October 1941): 798.

133 Robert Bud, *Penicillin: Triumph and Tragedy* (Oxford: Oxford University Press, 2007), 105.

134 Bud, *Penicillin: Triumph and Tragedy*, 105.

135 W. Michie and H.W.C. Bailie, 'A case of penicillin reaction', *The British Medical Journal* 1, 4398 (21 April 1945): 554.

136 Fletcher, 'Penicillin: A recent advance in chemotherapy', 799.

137 Fletcher, 'Penicillin: A recent advance in chemotherapy', 800.

138 Anonymous, 'Penicillin saves wounded soldiers', *The British Journal of Nursing* (September 1943): 104. If the use of penicillin for military personnel only was the subject of some debate, its use for gonorrhoea and syphilis caused anger. As Kevin Brown argues, sexually transmitted infections were considered by some to be self-inflicted wounds and by many to be the result of unacceptable, licentious behaviour. Brown, *Fighting Fit*, loc. 3514. The numbers of troops affected by venereal disease have been given by Harrison

in the Italian campaign as 51 per 1,000 in 1944, rising to 71 per 1,000 in 1945. Harrison, *Medicine and Victory*, 102. Despite the moral objections to the use of penicillin for sexually transmitted infections, the benefit to the war effort was seen as paramount. Treatment with sulphonamides for gonorrhoea could take up to 25 days and over 40 for syphilis; with penicillin this was reduced to 24 hours and four to five days, respectively. Harrison, *Medicine and Victory*, 107; Anonymous, 'Penicillin in the field', 738. Given the sheer numbers of those affected it would not have been possible for nursing staff to have ignored its presence, or to have not been in professional contact with those who were infected. Yet discussions of the care proffered to troops with VD are noticeable by their absence in personal testimonies. This is probably a result of notions of acceptable knowledge and issues of propriety for the nursing sisters. The purpose of this book is to consider the nurses' work and understanding of that work through their personal testimonies, this is largely the reason why VDs in general have not formed part of the wider discussion.

139 It seems that this was not entirely universal. In her oral history, Army Sister Mary Haddie Swan stated that penicillin was so precious that they used it only on their own troops in Normandy and not the German troops. Mary Haddie Swan, oral history by Lyn E. Smith, 26 October 1998, IWM Sound Archive 18571.

140 Anonymous, 'Penicillin for P.O.W.', *British Medical Journal* (7 October 1944): 484.

141 Anonymous, 'News from the nursing world: Professor Florey on penicillin', *Nursing Mirror and Midwives' Journal* (18 December 1943): 161.

142 Anonymous, 'Penicillin in the field', *The Lancet* (11 December 1943): 737. In her oral history interview, Ursula Dowling, a Red Cross nurse, discusses meeting Florey in the desert and his experiment on a patient with a gangrenous thigh. She described the effects as 'magic'. Ursula Dowling, oral history interview in 1986 by Rosemary Hart on behalf of the BBC. IWM oral history collection 9910.

143 H.E. Dale, 'Modern drugs: 3 – Penicillin', *Nursing Times* (27 November 1943): 883.

144 I.W.J. McAdam, J.P. Duguid and S.W. Challinor, 'Systemic administration of penicillin', *The Lancet* (9 September 1944): 336.

145 Anonymous, 'Penicillin in the treatment of war wounds', *Nursing Times* (8 January 1944): 19.

146 M.K.I. Harpin, 'Oral penicillin therapy in the nursing treatment of lobar pneumonia in the MEF'. This article was to be forwarded to the *Nursing Mirror and Midwives' Journal*, after approval of the General Headquarters. 25 February 1945, MMM QARANC uncatalogued archive.

147 Morris, 'The diary of a wartime nurse' (28 June1944), 116; Morris, *A Very Private Diary*, 99.

148 Morris, 'The diary of a wartime nurse' (8 October 1944), 148; Morris, *A Very Private Diary*, 130.
149 Bolton, *The Maturing Sun*, 131.
150 Gertrude Annie Cooper (née Ramsden), oral history interview by Margaret Skellern, 10 May 1994. Royal College of Nursing Oral History Archive, Edinburgh.
151 Dyer, 'When life was grey and scarlet', 62–3.
152 Salter, 'Long ago and far away', 147.
153 Luker, 'Preface', 14.
154 Anonymous, 'Penicillin in the field' 737.
155 Both the nursing and medical press published articles throughout 1944 and 1945 detailing the uses, dosages and administrative issues in penicillin. In both sets of professional journals the information given is strikingly similar, suggesting the expectation that both professions needed to learn about the drug and learn the same details. See, for example, Anonymous, 'Editorial: Penicillin treatment reviewed', *Nursing Times* (22 April 1944): 275; McAdam et al., 'Systemic administration of penicillin', 336–8; Anonymous, 'Penicillin: Indications for its use and methods of administration', *Nursing Mirror* (14 April 1945):16; Anonymous, 'Penicillin: Indications for its use and methods of administration', *The British Journal of Nursing* (April 1945): 39.
156 Sister Joan Peake, oral history by her son, Andrew Peake, 17 March 1993, 16. Princess Mary's Royal Air Force Nursing Service, Imperial War Museum, London 94/27/1. It is not absolutely clear at what point this was occurring. By 1944 there were reasonable quantities of penicillin being produced and it was therefore used instead of the sulpha drugs for many illnesses and injuries. If this was aa late as 1944, it is not clear why chemists were still producing crude penicillin. Peake's oral history is not particularly clear throughout in terms of timelines, so she could have been referring to earlier experiences in the desert. Kevin Brown identifies that the early researchers in Oxford did not have properly designed culture dishes either and that the team obtained biscuit tins, as well as petrol tins and bedpans, in order to grow the mould. Brown, *Fighting Fit*, loc. 3546.
157 Anonymous, 'Penicillin in the field', 738.
158 Toman, *An Officer and a Lady*, 131, 133.
159 Toman, *An Officer and a Lady*, 119.
160 Sandelowski, 'Venous envy'; Sandelowski, *Devices and Desires*; Toman, 'Blood work'; Cynthia Toman, '"Body work": Nurses and the delegation of medical technology at the Ottawa Civic Hospital, 1947–1972', *Canadian Journal of the History of Science, Technology and Medicine* 29, 2 (2006): 155–75.

5

Reasserting work, space and gender boundaries at the end of the Second World War

> When you come out of the Forces you will have eight weeks' leave in which to look round and take stock of your position … You have seen much, and you will bring to civilian life a broadened outlook. It may be that during your period of service you concentrated on one special branch of nursing work, while possibly losing touch with developments in other fields. Perhaps you held posts of great responsibility … While you have been away, those at home have had to carry on as best they could with sadly depleted ranks; so of one thing you can be certain: the civilian nursing service desperately needs your help … The vacancies are many, and if you have qualities of leadership, the big posts at home will be yours in the end; but do not be disappointed if, because you have held a position of authority in the field, you do not step straight away into a similar position at home. Not everyone who has risen to a matron-ship in His Majesty's Forces can hope for an immediate matron's post at home.[1]

These words, the RCN hoped, would galvanise demobilised military nurses to return to hospital practice. Its focus on what they could expect appears to have had the opposite effect. Many QAs had indeed worked in specialist areas, but within their work they had developed innovative practices, learnt new ways of working and established a more human-centred approach to patient care. The lack of understanding of these critical professional attributes would alienate the returning nurses and ultimately deny their talents to the British hospital service.

The vast majority of nurses whose stories have been used in *Negotiating Nursing* married and left the nursing profession, although some returned later in life when their children had grown up. A few went abroad to nurse, and at least two died young. The only testimony to identify both a satisfying professional career and a long and happy married life is that of Sister Catherine Hutchinson. Previous histories of allied military nurses have argued that they did not wish to return to hospital nursing because of its petty restrictions.[2] None of the testimonies in this book articulates this specifically. However, the evidence that is available suggests that hospital nursing was not a popular post-war choice.

The chapter considers the civilian world into which the QAs returned at the end of the war and explores the options they faced. It begins with the immediate aftermath of war and the opportunities for interesting and worthwhile work that would only exacerbate the nursing sisters' difficulties on demobilisation. This is followed by a consideration of the return to Britain and the options open for professional practice. It will be demonstrated that some nurses opted to return overseas, some entered work tangential to the nursing profession and some made careers in public health. A few remained in the military. The chapter then focuses on what was the main professional option for returning sisters – the crisis-ridden civilian hospital system. However, as it is argued, there were several constraints that made this unattractive. The nursing profession itself displayed a lack appreciation for the nurses' talents. Hospitals continued to demand complete devotion to the institution and its patients from female nursing staff, with the attendant need for nurses to live in.[3] Many nurses had married on active service overseas, or planned to marry at war's end. Unlike the social expectations of the men who became their husbands, for women, marriage was not expected to be combined with work outside the home, and this was only partly because of the professional boundaries placed on them. The reassertion of traditional gender rules post-war re-established discomfort with married women's work,[4] although in reality this never fell to pre-war figures.[5] It was considered highly desirable that marriage would rapidly lead to children.[6] Across the globe, the division of domestic labour was heavily focused on the wife, ostensibly compelling women to return to the home and remain there.[7] Finally, therefore, the chapter explores the choice of the majority: marriage, family and domesticity.

'An air of uncertainty'

> The bombs fell on Nagasaki and Hiroshima, August 15th 1945 became V.J. day and there were reverberations around the world. Reverberations were also felt at the 139 British General Hospital, Ranchi, Binar, India, where I was one of a contingent of Army nurses (QARANC) looking after the wounded from Burma. Excitement about the end of the war was followed by panic as an air of uncertainty prevailed.[8]

Anxieties about the end of the war resound through many of the nurses' testimonies. Sister Catherine Butland reflected on it being 'regretful that the seven months just past could not go in indefinitely, though very glad the fighting was over'.[9] However, for many nurses the war did not end in 1945, but as late as 1947. In the latter months and immediate post-war period, the needs of POWs, civilian inmates in concentration camps and the millions of starving people across the globe were to concentrate the minds and skills of some nursing sisters and provide further valuable work. In August 1946 Sister Ann Radloff was posted to a hospital train in Palestine. As she had been in the Army for over two years, she was designated 'Officer Commanding Train'. Although she admits that she had never 'felt less in command of anything' and that 'no-one took me seriously', her position, even nominally being in charge of anything but a hospital ward, contravened normal professional and gender rules and would have made Radloff's return to pre-war hierarchies challenging.[10] She was demobilised in 1947 after 'three years of exciting, terrifying and varying experiences. I look back in gratitude for the friendship and camaraderie of which I was part.'[11] Radloff was not to return to England permanently and later lived in South Africa, India and Nepal.[12]

Not all overseas postings were so savoured, especially those with the British Army of the Rhine (BAOR), although it is not clear if this is because of the work or the depressing nature of post-war Germany.[13] On 7 June 1945, Sister Mary Morris wrote in her diary: 'I have received my demobilisation number today, 56, whatever that means. I signed for the duration of the war, but in the medical corps that really means the duration of the emergency which is a different matter.'[14] There was no immediacy reflected in her demobilisation orders and in 1946 she was posted to Munster. Sister Elsie Gordon, also with the BAOR, wrote to the *Nursing Times* from post-war Berlin: 'the outlook is desolate and the atmosphere in Berlin very depressing. The sisters are glad of fairly frequent periods of leave.'[15] Morris herself maintained that her original posting to Munster with the 25th British General Hospital was the '"dead end" of B.A.O.R.'.[16] Following her marriage in October 1946, she was posted to Hamburg, where at least she and her new husband could be in the same city.[17] She was eventually demobilised in July 1947. Her diary entry for 27 July of that year reads, 'Today I am a civilian. It is so wonderful to be away from nursing and hospitals.'[18]

As the war in Europe drew to a close, the focus was switched to the continued hostilities in South-East Asia. Many sisters were sent to India to care for those men released from Changi and other Japanese camps.[19] One anonymous sister recalled that she was nursing men whom she had previously nursed in Italy; for some it had been a very long war.[20] Sister C.M.S. Baker's final posting in September 1945 was to care for released British POWs:

> We had to cope with men, after years of deprivation, cut off from news of family and home, suffering from malnutrition and the effects of cruelty, who now had to adjust to a normal way of living. Some hid their food in their lockers ... in case ... [ellipses in the original] some wept uncontrollably at times and some wanted to stand to attention if spoken to ... We let the patients do their own thing ... We had no routine, treated them as gently as possible and accepted some eccentricities.[21]

Other nurses were posted to care for the liberated civilian inmates of Nazi concentration camps. It is the experiences of nurses who were part of the liberation and later rehabilitation of the inmates at Bergen-Belsen concentration camp that provide some of the most traumatic narratives of early post-war nursing work and illustrate the impending difficulties that these nurses would have on return to Britain.[22] Sister Mary Bond was posted with 29th British General Hospital to Belsen in May 1945, by which time 'I was proud to be a senior Sister with many added responsibilities'.[23] Bond was placed in charge of one of the hospital blocks at the camp, but she 'felt inadequate in [her] capacity as a nurse to even try to counteract in any way the atrocities they had suffered'.[24] Key to her ability to support those in her care were her fundamental nursing skills that she had learnt in her training, combined with the shifts in work and nurse–patient relationship boundaries developed in the war:

> Also under my supervision in Square Eleven was a ward full of patients suffering from Cancrum Oris – extensive ulceration of the mucus lining of the cheeks due to lack of mastication and malnutrition. The patients developed holes in their cheeks, and the tongue could be seen moving as they spoke. Even though I had learnt of this condition in nurse training, this was the first time I had ever encountered it when practicing. Such was the lack of control over the mouth area that feeding was made very difficult. After each feed we had to wash the mouth, cleanse the surrounding ulcerated areas, and spray them with penicillin.[25]

Sisters Myrtle Beardwell and Molly Silva Jones of the British Red Cross were amongst the first nurses to enter the camp in April 1945, joining Lieutenant Colonel Johnston, RAMC with 32 CCS. Silva Jones described how the patients' cries for food, ''will haunt the ears of those who heard them for a long time to come'.[26] She was 'Stirred [with] an increased desire to help; nothing we could do was enough to attempt to restore these sub-humans to some measure of mental and physical health.'[27] In a letter to the *Nursing Times* Sister B.B., with the 2nd Army, wrote, 'Soon we shall be leaving Belsen, with no sorrow and no regrets. We shall remember it only as a sad, harrowing experience.'[28]

Despite the nurses' doubts of their abilities to help the survivors, they were considered by the senior medical staff to be the most critical members of the team. Lieutenant Colonel F.M. Lipscombe, RAMC, also with 32 CCS, maintained that 'Better results might have been obtained with a larger staff of skilled nurses.'[29] Johnston even admitted in one report that 'medical skill is of secondary importance' and that the most important resource requirement was nurses.[30] Nursing staff were integral to the work at Belsen as they eased the suffering and, alongside relief workers of all nationalities, worked to restore life and humanity into the camp's survivors.[31] The importance of the nurses' work rendered their skills essential to the liberation of the inmates and created a collegiality with their male colleagues that perhaps even surpassed previous war work.[32] Other nurses found that they were now not only the colleagues of the medical profession, but their leaders.

Barbara Mortimer cites the letter home by Sister Mary Copeland in which she described how she was 'now running a building with 180 patients who are being looked after by ten German orderlies, three German sisters and two German doctors, and I might add it is not an unpleasant position to be in, that of supervising doctors, and telling them what to do, quite apart from them being Germans'.[33] This reversal of professional order was also described by Sister Mary Sands, a QA who arrived, probably with 32 CCS, soon after the liberation.[34] The nursing sisters had significant autonomy in their duties. Sister Kathleen Elvidge wrote home: 'There is one English doctor to each square of five blocks, so as you can imagine we don't see much of her. Then we have some Belgian medical students who also help, I've got two assigned to my block.'[35] The official sanctioning of male doctors and medical students being placed under female nurses was a considerable alteration of normal gender and professional rules. For these nursing sisters and others from across all war zones, the multiple ways and situations in which they had been placed in authority, given autonomy and had developed new ways of working would be lost in the return to peace and pre-war hospital hierarchies. For some nurses the end of the war offered an extension of interesting, if harrowing work, but there was a growing 'normality' that was felt by some even as they returned to Britain's military hospitals.

Return to normality?

Sister Penny Salter's reaction to her return home from active service overseas was one of boredom and a lack of commonality with those who had stayed behind:

> Arriving back in the United Kingdom was quite an anti-climax, and I found on meeting my parents and relatives again I was quite lost, as if we had nothing in common anymore. Also I was not interested in anything or anyone pertaining to the family, as for Christmas in the immediate future, that was the last thing I wanted, everyone going out of their way to please me made me feel worse than ever, all I wanted was to get away and be myself … However, one morning in Piccadilly Circus, outside the well-known store of Swan and Edgars, who should I bump into but my surgeon friend Colonel Van Rensburg and his wife from Kenya – It was quite extraordinary for amongs't [*sic*] our conversation on mentioning my feelings he soon assured me by saying this was quite a normal reaction, many people felt the same – not to worry, it would soon wear off. I wondered![36]

Like many returning Army nursing reservists, Salter had a period of demobilisation leave, after which she states, 'it was quite a relief when I eventually received my posting orders to report to the Military Hospital at Stover Park in Devon'.[37] Too soon she realised that military nursing in a British hospital was not as interesting as an overseas posting: 'The work itself I found most boring, mainly because it was so dull, including medical boards and the chronic sick from Burma.'[38] The boredom did not abate, and on 1 May 1947, Salter left England to join the Medical and Nursing Service of Rhodesia (now Zimbabwe).[39] During the war, nursing sisters of the British Army had been posted to hostile zones in which the hospitals were 'filled to the brim with unceasing casualties, terrible wounds and shocking conditions'.[40] It was no surprise that they struggled to find satisfaction in positions and work that echoed pre-war professional life.[41] Overseas service had been an adventure and a heroic endeavour; nursing back in Britain was mundane and firmly relocated within the gendered and professional expectations of the female nurse and women more generally.[42]

Sister Jessie Wilson was sent home in 1943 after several periods of ill health. Following her recuperation, she managed to organise a posting to work at a hospital in the Midlands with her old matron from the Middle East. Excited about seeing her again and reminiscing, her memoir demonstrates the frustration of many of the returning nurses when she wrote: 'Matron told me things were very different from the way things were run in the Middle East and one had to readjust one's ideas.'[43] Sister P.M. Dyer returned to Britain to be posted to Aldershot Military Hospital in Surrey:

> Those first few weeks back in civilised surroundings were like commencing training days all over again. The greatest tragedy of all appeared to be that everyone, bound up in their efficiency, had become quite mechanised and the art of a sense of humour seemed to have disappeared … the greatest hardship was to be told by a senior Sister how to carry out a particular job and with complete demureness one answer [*sic*] 'Yes Sister', 'No Sister', 'Certainly Sister'.[44]

It was clear to those nursing sisters who had experienced overseas service that their colleagues who had remained in Britain had little idea of the lives they had led during the war. The RCN recommended its demobbed members to be realistic about their talents and abilities to work in civilian hospitals.[45] In reality, it was their colleagues on the home front who had been 'left behind' in the scientific and nursing developments that had occurred in the midst of battle.[46] In May 1945, the *British Journal of Nursing* had published a statement from Major-General Norman T. Kirk, the Surgeon-General of the US Army. In it he maintained that 'the Army Nurse is living five years ahead of the Nursing Profession. She is handling new drugs, applying new treatments and working with the surgeons who are making history in medical circles during this war. She is gaining experience years ahead of her civilian opportunities. The urgent need for nurses continues to be critical.'[47] Notwithstanding such sentiments, military nurses returned to British hospitals where they were expected to follow nursing regimes they had abandoned on active service. Even military hospitals in Britain would not countenance the continued autonomous ways of practice of those who had experienced overseas postings. The stifling of returning military nurses' ingenuity and abilities to improvise was a forerunner to the realities of civilian practice. Some nurses could not and would not accept these options. For a fortunate few, the chance to remain in the military, or join the Colonial Office and return to overseas service, meant that they could pursue the autonomy of practice they had so relished during the war.

Returning abroad

At the end of the war, the 12,000-strong QA force was reduced to its 624 peacetime numbers.[48] Those who had joined as regulars before 1938 could remain in the service, but the reservists were demobilised. Sister Vera Jones wrote to her parents from India on 29 December 1944, informing them that she had applied to join the regulars of the QAs, with the full support of her principal matron.[49] Less than one quarter of the 455 nurses who applied to join as a regular at the end of the war could be accepted.[50] For those who were recruited or retained in the service, the opportunities of overseas postings and the professional status afforded by commissioned officer rank were highly attractive and some women had important military nursing careers. Sister Monica Johnson, later Dame Monica Golding, had served with the BEF and then in Egypt during the war, and was posted to India as Principal Matron between 1946 and 1948. She became Director of Army Nursing Services of the QARANC in the early 1950s.[51] Sister Margot Turner, later Dame Margot Turner, became Director of Army Nursing Services of QARANC in 1964.[52] Turner had been posted to Malaya as the Japanese invaded in December 1941 and spent the rest of the war in Japanese internment camps.[53] Despite this, on her release in October 1945, she wanted to return to work and within 18 months was on active service again.[54] Nevertheless, given the quota of the peacetime nursing service, the prospect of such an interesting professional life was limited to only a very few.

There was also the option to join the TANS, and several nursing sisters did so, though little is known about their post-war lives.[55] A few Second World War nurses were lucky enough to combine both public health work and travel abroad, although the evidence is sparse, and they appear to have been only a very small minority of the cohort. For example, G. Padfield, who had been a reservist, found a post-war career as a health visitor for the Libyan government.[56] Sally Hepworth joined the Foreign and Commonwealth Office and was posted to Malaya.[57] Sister Marjorie Hunt admitted that she 'couldn't settle down after the war' and went to Rhodesia in 1946 following an interview with the Society for Professional and Business Women.[58] Others secured work in careers tangential to nursing. Jane Patterson, who had been Chief Principal Matron in India until 1947, took up a post as the Warden of the International House for Students, the residence for those nurses from abroad studying post-registration courses in London.[59] Such opportunities were limited, however, and with the vacancies for hospital nursing across the country in the thousands, demobbed military nurses were called upon to take up these posts.

A professional future?

The promised new welfare state needed more nurses, health visitors and social workers.[60] The hospitals of the NHS founded on 5 July 1948 would need a skilled nursing workforce.[61] Sister Catherine Hutchinson was demobbed in December 1946. When she was on demobilisation leave, she read an article in the *Readers' Digest* about the work at East Grinstead Hospital. Later, on seeing an advert in the *Nursing Times* for a year's course in 'Burns' nursing, plastic surgery and jaw injuries', she applied.[62] On 14 June 2001, she wrote that 'Many of the war-time burnt air crew were still there, receiving treatment (McIndoe was still there doing his pioneering work). With them as a group, I fell in love, married one, worked in the hospital for 23 years and lived happily ever after.'[63] Sister Helen Luker also returned to hospital nursing. She was first appointed as the tutor for the preliminary training school of the Nightingale School of Nursing at St Thomas' Hospital, where she herself had trained. Later she went to St Thomas' country hospital, Hydestile, as Sister-in-Charge. Luker was still in post when, in May 1957, she suffered a seizure and died.[64]

Although Luker's career ended in her early death, both she and Hutchinson had secured work that would allow a level of autonomy reminiscent of their war careers. As is discussed in Chapter 3 of this volume, nurses were obliged to accept harassment and unwanted sexual advances at East Grinstead Hospital, but they were also given professional and clinical responsibilities that were unusual in hospital practice. It is significant that amongst all the nurses' testimonies, it is these two who identify their post-war careers, given that they both had the opportunity for professionally satisfying work within hospital nursing. Information regarding other nurses who, on return from active service, chose hospital nursing practice is very limited. Penny Starns identifies problems related to the recruitment and retention of nurses in general, which were, she argues, due to the arch-regimentation of hospital life in response to the increased militarisation of the nursing profession.[65] Whilst this may have some credence, demobbed nursing sisters were used to the form-filling and rank-awareness of the military and are unlikely to have been particularly alarmed by this. Rather, as Barbara Mortimer maintains, it was 'the prospect of returning to nursing in a traditional, hierarchical hospital setting' rather than a new militarisation of hospitals that 'was not appealing'.[66]

The nursing profession at home failed to appreciate the demobbed sisters' clinical knowledge and new methods of patient engagement. Military nurses had developed a knowledge base related to post-operative care, intensive care treatments and diagnostic awareness. They were used to practising with levels of autonomy that were not permitted and that in some cases were not even acknowledged in post-war hospitals.[67] It was not unknown for ex-military nurses to get patients out of bed post-operatively, only for civilian nurses to put them back again.[68] Such dissonant attitudes to nursing care frustrated the ex-military nurses and angered the civilian ones. As Starns argues, 'the war on the wards continued'.[69] Civilian nurses expected their demobbed military nursing colleagues to return to civilian work and abide by its rules, just as they had done before the war.[70]

Sisters Catherine Butland and Vera Jones were both unsure of the opportunities for nursing sisters in the post-war period. Jones wrote to her parents on 30 September 1944 of her thoughts about joining the regular QAs after the war:

> It will not be easy to find good positions in civil hospitals, for while we are away overseas, other nurses are being trained and they in their turn will seek trained nurse positions. The new Rushcliffe rates of pay will draw many more girls to nursing from now onwards and the hospitals should never again suffer that acute shortage of staff as during my training.[71]

Jones was wrong about staff shortages and the 'draw' of improved pay.[72] The Rushcliffe Committee may have increased nurses' salaries,[73] but the 40 per cent rise in the cost of living between 1940 and 1943 all but obliterated the improvements. Nurses were no better off.[74] She was, however, right in her summation of the difficulties in finding good positions in hospitals. Butland was equally unsure of her future, believing that her skills as an Army nursing sister would not be useful in civilian practice, the two jobs being so different. Furthermore, she maintained that those who had stayed at home and those who had been demobilised early would get the most 'enviable vacancies', leaving those still on active service overseas with the least attractive jobs.[75] Her prescience in this matter demonstrates an awareness of the difficulties that nurses returning from war would face – not because the skills they had developed would not be valuable to the new scientific management of patients, for example, in the provision of penicillin regimes, but because they were not wanted.

An editorial in the *Nursing Times* on 19 January 1946 offered this blunt assessment of demobbed nursing sisters: 'Even though they may be obviously abler women, many committees of management will not have the courage to appoint them.'[76] Butland's later comments suggest an acknowledgement of the difference in status between military and civilian nurses that would fuel intra-professional rivalry and jealousy.

Butland's memoir ends with, 'Now I was no longer a member of the Q.A.I.M.N.S. but just a civilian nurse, and my thoughts were identical to what they were when I first received my calling up papers – I wonder what the future will hold?'[77] The use of the word 'just' is intuitive. There is an almost fatalistic appreciation that, as a civilian nurse, her professional status would reduce and that the work would once again be mundane. Indeed, not only did hospitals struggle to recruit returning nurses, they struggled to recruit nurses at all.

According to Susan McGann and colleagues, in March 1945 there were 11,000 hospital nursing vacancies.[78] Three years later, in 1948, the total shortfall was somewhere between 40,000 and 50,000.[79] In December 1948, the *British Journal of Nursing* published highlights of a House of Lords debate on the nursing shortage. In the opinion of Lord Crook, it stated, the 'actual number of vacancies for nurses was 33,000, though to meet the present-day shortage 50,000 nurses, and no less [*sic*], were required. The efficiency of the Health Service would depend upon the number of nurses obtained.'[80] In a letter to the editor of *The Times* on 16 May 1945, Gladys Carter and Evelyn Pearce wrote that 'The shortage of nurses causes concerns to Ministers and public alike and threatens to bring the hospital services to a full stop.'[81]

British hospitals were struggling not only to recruit returning military nurses, but also new students. The status of nurses in training, Carter argued, was dubious, and calling them students 'camouflaged' their uncertain position. This would, she maintained, continue to create difficulties in the aspiration to establish nursing as a desirable profession.[82] Even Dame Katharine Jones thought that some of the criticisms in the press and media about the pettiness of hospital life were 'not without some justification'.[83] References to nurses as workers, 'ancillary to medicine', did little to raise the profession's prestige and were even disliked by doctors.[84] The profession's attempts to persuade young women to enter nursing with promises of its 'marvellous opportunities for service' may have been 'true enough and the argument is therefore powerful. But it has one blemish and it is fatal. It does not persuade those women it aims at persuading.'[85]

If the health system as a whole needed the demobbed nurses to resume their nursing careers, hospitals themselves did little to encourage them. Most hospitals continued to advertise for nurses who would be required to 'live in' and identified the residential emoluments in support of this expectation.[86] The *Nursing Times* ran a series of articles from 1945 on the matter of 'living in', but advice that non-residential posts should have been made available seem to have been ignored. On 11 August 1945, the editorial of the *Nursing Times* argued that the question of a non-resident staff nurse and ward sister was 'a vital matter or the future of the recruitment problem'.[87] In December 1945, the *Nursing Times* was even calling for student nurses to be allowed to live away from the hospital.[88] In February 1946, the particular problem of the needs and wishes of demobbed nurses to live independent lives was raised,[89] but there is nothing to suggest that any of these demands were met. The blame cannot be laid entirely at the door of the profession.

According to an editorial on 17 November 1945, Aneurin Bevan stated that 'all had *accepted the principle that trained nursing staff should be readily permitted to live out* ... Unfortunately the proposed increase in the living out allowance is not sufficient.'[90] Furthermore, whilst demobilised medical officers were provided with funded post-graduate training, the same options were not available to the demobbed nurses.[91] Even the *Nursing Times* could see that such policies conspired to keep returning military nurses from hospital practice and would in turn stymie educational and professional advancements.[92] Yet rather than addressing such inequities, the profession turned to women from overseas and the very young to staff the wards of the country.

Recruitment drives in former colonies to find women willing to train as nurses were established in the late 1940s, but many would be channelled into the lower-grade state enrolled nurse (SEN) training that had been created in the war years to alleviate nursing shortages. This move supported the class superiority of the registered nurse and created de facto racial segregation in the profession. Many of these nurses realised too late that the SEN qualification had no currency anywhere else in the world.[93] Nurse training schools also developed 'Nurse Cadet' schemes to bring young girls into the sphere of the nursing workforce before they could find alternative work on leaving school[94] – a scheme that Penny Starns asserts was little more than child exploitation.[95] The Ministry of Health did not agree to the return of compulsory educational entry criteria into nursing until 1959.[96] The consequence of such a policy was that nurse training schools were free to recruit girls with only two 'O' Levels that could be taken serially. Thus, apart from in the prestigious teaching hospitals, nurse training programmes and, ultimately, the hospitals of Britain were replete with academically weak students.[97]

In order to recruit more experienced staff to the healthcare system, the profession then focused on those men who had been released from the forces. These former RAMC orderlies were offered shortened training without the requirement to live in, to try to arrest the growing numbers of vacancies in hospitals.[98] Although these men, like female nurses recruited from the former colonies, were usually in the lower ranks of nursing, male nurses were paid a higher salary than their female counterparts. This understandably caused significant consternation, including within the RCN itself.[99] Male nurses were therefore neither the cheaper option, like nurses from the former colonies and cadet nurses, nor were they likely to be as malleable. Nevertheless, despite the attractive conditions of service offered to ex-military orderlies, recruitment from their ranks was also limited. These strategies that failed to attract experienced nurses and favoured cheap and frequently less able candidates meant that in order to protect patients, ward sisters had to assert careful discipline. The authoritarian regime did not appeal to those nurses returning from overseas postings. Most simply married.

'Your nursing days are over, sweetheart'

After the chaos of the war, the nation wanted to return to stability and most women returned to the home, marriage and family.[100] Although the marriage bar in nursing had been lifted during the war, it was all but re-established in its aftermath.[101] That is not to say that it was impossible to combine the two, as the discussion of Catherine Hutchinson's post-war career above demonstrates. Nevertheless, despite the shortage of nurses, many hospitals created significant obstacles to the employment of those who were married. Most of the nurses whose testimonies have been used for this book married men they had met on active service, thus denying their skills to the British health system. Sister Florence Hardy joined the QAs during the Second Front and was posted to France, Belgium and Germany. She was demobbed soon after the end of the war and spent some time as a private nurse and then worked in a London hospital. In 1948 she married an Army colonel whom she had met in Belgium, at which point, like many other women, she left work and settled into a domestic life.[102] Sister Joan Carr was not demobbed until 1948, having joined the QAs late in the war. In the immediate post-war period she was posted to Gibraltar, which she said was an interesting time. On return to Britain she worked for a short time in the theatres at her local hospital and then married in 1950.[103] Morris met her husband, Malcolm, on 7 April 1945 and married him on 12 October in the same year. Her diary states, 'I know that I love him and will marry him.'[104] Sister Daphne Ingram left the QARANC in 1947 and married a gunner officer whom she had met in her first year in Hong Kong.[105] Sister Joyce Parry Ffoulkes married in May 1943, after which both she and her new husband returned briefly to their military work before demobilisation. On the last page of her edited diary she wrote, 'Now I am facing the other way and beginning my real life.'[106]

Sister Betty Evans married in May 1945, but was immediately sent back to Holland with her unit. At the end of the war, she joined her husband for a while in Poona and they returned to England together in 1946, at which point Evans left nursing because she wanted a family, 'and naturally I had to be in civilian life to have a family'.[107] Sister Betty Parkin's memoir recalls her new husband, Stanley's, comment upon their marriage, '"Your nursing days are over, sweetheart", my husband said as we sat for the first time in our own sitting-room with the windows opened wide onto flower-filled beds.'[108] Toman argues with reference to the Canadian nursing sisters that the return to domesticity was partly because professional options were so limited. As Evans' and Parkin's recollections suggest, neither the general public nor individual husbands expected wives to work after marriage. The reasons for nursing sisters not to return to hospital nursing post-marriage were therefore more complex than limited professional opportunities.

Military nurses had been awarded officer status, with its associated privileges and salary, but on demobilisation that status disappeared.[109] The position of nurses was untenable. Their lives were severely curtailed by being required to live in, often in similar conditions to the student nurses under their charge and with very little money.[110] Even experienced ward sisters could not afford to buy their own homes, nor could they necessarily provide for their old age:[111] 'because they said it was a vocation, you know, it wasn't a job, so you didn't get much money, you got your keep'.[112] The nursing and medical press called for married women to be able to continue to hold senior posts in the nursing profession, a move that it was argued 'might help to ventilate the cloistered atmosphere'. Such calls were not heeded.[113] The ongoing and unresolved debates about living in meant that even those experienced demobbed nurses who were willing to accept the social criticism directed at women who combined work and marriage could not always find positions. In 1945 the Minister for Health argued that 'there should be no bar on the employment of married women nurses, including those who desire to live out, provided they can give the service required by the hospital. Married student nurses should also be allowed to continue their training.'[114] In view of the gendered assumption that a married woman could not look after her husband and give appropriate service to her patients, is likely that matrons used the 'provided they can give the service required by the hospital' to deny them employment. Despite knowing that choosing marriage meant forgoing a professional life, women, including nurses across the country, chose marriage.

The desire to return to 'normal' family life was, according to Richard Bessel and Dirk Schumann, even more important to the nations which had been affected by the Second World War than those of the First World War. That earlier conflict may have been brutal and dehumanising, but it did not witness the destruction of whole swathes of the civilian population in the mass bombing of cities or the genocide of European Jewry.[115] How could such memories be managed, or understood, how could the guilt of even knowing what happened be assuaged?[116] Better to bury that knowledge. The problem for nurses and other women workers was that the normality that was sought was one based in the male hegemony of the mid-twentieth century. Normality meant women being returned to the home, childbirth and child rearing, whilst men regained a sense of self through civilian work.[117]

The war had temporarily extended women's access to work outside the home, but this access was for the duration only, and was fraught with complex gendered contradictions.[118] Women in Britain had been expected to be active citizens for the war effort, but to remain feminine.[119] They were expected to 'keep the home fires burning', but their homes were bombed. They were expected to be generous to fighting men, but to be so in a way that did not contravene expected sexual and social mores.[120] Nevertheless, although women had only been 'filling in the gaps' whilst the men went to war,[121] across the globe many found even this contingent participation in the public world emancipating.[122] The cessation of hostilities witnessed an end to the gender-bending attitudes that had been tolerated during the war and a reassertion of traditional social mores.

At war's end, demobilised women were expected to return to the home, to care for their husbands and raise their children.[123] The men, however, re-established themselves in the jobs that they had 'donated' to their womenfolk whilst they had been away fighting. Propaganda to encourage the reinstatement of traditional family life was extensive. Official texts such as *Rebuilding Family Life in the Post-War World* quickly reasserted the regard for women who stayed at home.[124] Arguments were made that there had been an increase in juvenile delinquency amongst the young because mothers had been out at work during the war. The only way to reduce delinquency was for women to return to the home.[125] Dr Eliot Slater, one of the contributors to the pamphlet, was even more stark: 'It needs at least two people to run a house, one to earn the money, the other to look after the house.'[126] Many ordinary members of the public also wished to restore pre-war social constructs that vilified all women,[127] including the educated and professional, who tried to combine marriage and work.[128]

New domestic appliances and technologies may have been advertised as methods to free the women of Britain from the burden of domestic drudgery, but the work remained women's work.[129] According to Harold Smith, surveys conducted in the latter months of the war, showed that only about 25 per cent of women who had been employed in factories during the war wanted to stay in work. Most wished to get married and have children.[130] Given that factory work was monotonous and unpleasant, to identify this as a trend for all women is simplistic. Yet the expectation was so pervasive that even women's magazines heralded the return to the home and hearth as the normal and desirable space for women.[131] Certainly the historiography of post-war women's lives suggests that many women were happy to return to the home after the chaos of war.[132]

The Mass Observation Unit's own assessment was that service women, having in many cases experienced true adventure, would be less likely to wish to return to domestic life.[133] Nevertheless, even women who had taken on some of the most dangerous wartime work, such as those in the SOE, married quickly post-war and settled into domestic routine and traditional home lives.[134] Ali Haggart's oral history study of housewives from the post-war period identifies women who were glad to return to the home and relished their time raising their children, even if their relationships with their husbands were not always a positive experience.[135] In *Reconstructing Women's Wartime Lives*, Penny Summerfield expresses a level of surprise at the number of women who maintained they were pleased to return to a more traditional role of home and hearth, with 38 of the 42 women interviewed marrying post-war.[136] Summerfield acknowledges the belief of Marxist feminists in the 1970s and early 1980s that these women were expressing a 'false consciousness' or 'collusion' in their desire to return home,[137] but suggests that such an attitude towards the generation of women who returned to 'normal' civilian life after the Second World War is unnecessarily pejorative. Women wanted to marry and have a family.[138] The critical issue was that, unlike the men they married, the social pressure to not work outside the home once married was significant. In the absence of contraception that enabled the women themselves to control child-birth, the birth rate rose rapidly.[139] With the closing of nurseries at the end of hostilities, many women had no choice but to return to the home to care for their children.[140]

Although working-class women had invariably worked during their marriage out of necessity, middle-class women did not. Not working, therefore, became a social aspiration for women of the respectable working class and lower middle class. Deborah Montgomerie maintains that 'Women homemakers, actual and potential, were reverenced and praised within the wartime iconography of femininity.'[141] It was thus not difficult to cultivate this into a trope of arch-domesticity in the post-war era as men were demobilised and needed 'their' jobs back. The complex interplay of social expectation, economic necessity and romantic love played into this ideology and women returned to the domestic space and marriage. Nursing had long offered social mobility to women from the lower middle class or respectable working class. Having gained social mobility through nursing and joined the middle class, they were expected to follow its codes and leave the profession on marriage; married middle-class women did not work.[142] As with previous generations, experienced nurses were therefore lost to the profession.

Conclusion

The final months of the war provided nursing sisters with some of the most challenging work of their wartime careers. Restoring the liberated inmates of Bergen-Belsen to a semblance of humanity and rehabilitating men who had been POWs of the Japanese demanded exemplary clinical skills and also methods of patient engagement that would rarely have been encountered on the wards of British hospitals pre-war. Despite the valuable professional skills that active service overseas and this war's-end work had engendered, few demobbed nurses had the chance to support the development of the profession in the post-war British hospital system. The reason for the limited acknowledgement of these new and important nursing methods in hospitals has previously been levelled at the profession itself. The demobbed nurses could not or would not re-engage with such a rigid system. The nurses' testimonies used in this book suggest a more complex depiction of post-war opportunities.

Hospitals did not encourage living out and, despite government claims that opportunities for independent living should be available, nurses' salaries were not commensurate with private home rental and the government would not provide additional allowances. Furthermore, post-graduate training opportunities for demobbed medical officers were not matched for nursing sisters, thus precluding them from developing themselves for senior positions. Finally, many nurses did not return to the profession because they wanted to marry, or had already married on active service. Some hospitals certainly made recruitment very difficult for married women, but the nation more widely wanted women to return to the home and raise families. Demobilised nursing sisters were therefore caught in the interstices of traditionalist hospital regimes with long hours, erratic off-duty and limited options for living independently and post-war conservatism that demanded that women should marry and bear children. In the absence of nurseries, and faced with the prospect of the double burden of home and professional work, many women, including nurses, had no choice but to return to the home and stay there.

Notes

1 The Advisory Service of the Royal College of Nursing, 'The re-settlement of nurses: Back to civilian life' (London: H. and Co., December 1945), 1.

2 Penny Starns, 'Fighting militarism? British nursing during the Second World War', in Roger Cooter, Mark Harrison and Steve Sturdy (eds), *War, Medicine and Modernity* (Stroud: Sutton Publishing, 1998), 197; Mary Sarnecky, *A History of the US Army Nurse Corps* (Philadelphia, PA: University of Pennsylvania Press, 1999), 280; Penny Starns, *Nurses at War: Women on the Frontline, 1939–45* (Stroud: Sutton Publishing, 2000), 152–8; Cynthia Toman, *An Officer and a Lady: Canadian Military Nursing and the Second World War* (Vancouver: University of British Columbia Press, 2007), 184–7; Nicola Tyrer, *Sisters in Arms: British Army Nurses Tell their Story* (London: Phoenix, 2008), 303–4.

3 There were debates in the nursing press related to the need for student nurses to live in, but not those who were qualified. Nevertheless, comments such as 'sickness is much more prevalent amongst non-residents', do suggest an antipathy towards nurses living away from the hospital. V.E. Darley, 'Living out is *not* such an advantage', *Nursing Mirror* (23 March 1946): 424; Anonymous, 'Living out and living in', *Nursing Mirror* (2 March 1946): 361–2.

4 Sonya O. Rose, *Which People's War? National Identity and Citizenship in Britain, 1939–1945* (Oxford: Oxford University Press, 2003, Kindle edition), loc. 3830.

5 Sue Bruley, *Women in Britain since 1900* (Basingstoke: Palgrave Macmillan, 1999), 118.

6 Margaret Hadley Jackson, 'Causes and significance of the dwindling family', in Sir James Marchant (ed.), *Rebuilding Family Life in the Post-War World: An Enquiry with Recommendations* (London: Odhams Press, 1945), 89.

7 Sarah Burke Odland, 'Unassailable motherhood, ambivalent domesticity: The construction of maternal identity in Ladies' Home Journal in 1946', *Journal of Communication Inquiry* 34, 1 (2010): 61–84.

8 C.M.S. Baker, 'Aftermath of war, September 1945', Imperial War Museum Private Papers (hereafter IWM) Documents 6341. It should be noted that the Queen Alexandra's Imperial Military Nursing Service did not actually change its name to the Queen Alexandra's Royal Army Nurse Corps (QARANC) until 1 February 1948. Juliet Piggott, *Queen Alexandra's Royal Army Nurse Corps* (London: Leo Cooper, 1975), 86.

9 Catherine M. Butland, 'Army sisters in battledress or the chosen few or follow fate', 89, MMM QARANC/PE/1/74/BUTL Box 8. The seven months refers to her time with the No. 1 Mobile Military Hospital which she and four colleagues had rejoined the previous Christmas. Cynthia Toman identifies the dissonance that many nurses felt at the end of the war. They were, she argues, glad the war was over, but sad to return to lives that would never be as exciting again. Toman, *An Officer and a Lady*, 167.

10 Ann Radloff, 'Going to Gooseberry Beach: Travels and adventures of a nursing sister', 27, IWM Documents 147.

11 Radloff, 'Going to Gooseberry Beach', 30.

12 The information relating to Radloff's later life is not available in her memoir. Although the contents page identifies that these travels are considered in part 2 of the memoir, the IWM archivists are not aware of these later chapters. There is no second part to her memoir in their collection. It is not therefore known whether her travels were as a professional nurse, as a wife or in another capacity.

13 The BAOR was an employer not only of nurses, but of women more generally. The need for women to participate in post-war reconstruction overseas created work in the British zone in Germany. Although many welcomed this work as a change to the confines of their British home life, they were placed in low-level clerical jobs, where there was little autonomy or relinquishment of servitude to their male bosses. Ruth Easingwood, '"I was merely a shorthand typist": British women at work in the British zone of occupied Germany, 1945–1949', *Women's History Magazine* 67 (2011): 20–7.

14 Mary Morris, 'The diary of a wartime nurse' (7 June 1945), 198, IWM Documents 4850; Mary Morris, *A Very Private Diary: A Nurse in Wartime*, ed. Carol Acton (London: Weidenfeld and Nicolson, 2014), 171.

15 J. Elsie Gordon, 'With the BAFO and BAOR – 4: In the depressing city of Berlin', *Nursing Times* (8 December 1945): 158.

16 Morris, 'The diary of a wartime nurse' (21 July 1945); Morris, *A Very Private Diary*, 257.

17 Morris, 'The diary of a wartime nurse' (16 June 1947).

18 Morris, 'The diary of a wartime nurse' (27 July 1947); Morris, *A Very Private Diary*, 281.

19 Cecelia Helen Burnette Christie, oral history interview by Conrad Wood, 25 March 1993, IWM Sound Archive 13121.

20 Anonymous, oral history interview by Conrad Wood in 1998, IWM Sound Archive 18451.

21 Baker, 'Aftermath of war, September 1945', 2–3.

22 For detailed discussions on the work of nurses at Bergen-Belsen Concentration Camp, see for example, Jane Brooks, '"Uninterested in anything except food": Nurse feeding work with the feeding the liberated

inmates of Bergen-Belsen', *Journal of Clinical Nursing* 21 (2012): 2958–65; Jane Brooks, '"The nurse stoops down … for me": Nursing the liberated persons at Bergen-Belsen', in Jane Brooks and Christine Hallett (eds), *One Hundred Years of Nursing Wartime Practices, 1854–1953* (Manchester: Manchester University Press, 2015). There are a range of texts about the liberation of Bergen-Belsen, including the medical aspects. See especially Jo Reilly, David Cesarani, Tony Kushner and Colin Richmond (eds), *Belsen in History and Memory* (London: Frank Cass, 1997); Ben Flanagan and Donald Bloxham (eds), *Remembering Belsen: Eyewitnesses Record the Liberation* (London: Vallentine Mitchell, 2005); Ben Shephard, *After Daybreak: The Liberation of Belsen, 1945* (London, Pimlico, 2005); Suzanne Bardgett and David Cesarani (eds), *Belsen 1945, New Historical Perspectives* (London: Vallentine Mitchell, 2006); Leslie Hardman and Cecily Goodman, *The Survivors: The Story of the Belsen Remnant* (London: Vallentine Mitchell, 2009); Mark Celinscak, 'At war's end: Allied forces at Bergen-Belsen' [unpublished PhD thesis] (Toronto: York University, 2012).

23 Mary Bond, *Wartime Experiences from the Midnight Sun to Belsen* (Cardigan: E.L. Jones and Son, 1994), 47.

24 Bond, *Wartime Experiences from the Midnight Sun to Belsen*, 47–8.

25 Bond, *Wartime Experiences from the Midnight Sun to Belsen*, 48.

26 Molly Silva Jones, 'From a diary written in Belsen' (1945), 4, IWM Documents 9550.

27 Jones, 'From a diary written in Belsen', 2.

28 Sister B.B., 'Nursing in Belsen Camp', *Nursing Times* (14 July 1945): 204.

29 F.M. Lipscombe, 'Medical aspects of Belsen concentration camp', *The Lancet* (8 September 1945): 314.

30 J.A.D. Johnston, 'Administrative report – Belsen Concentration Camp', 3 (c. June 1945), IWM Documents 10541.

31 Brooks, '"The nurse stoops down … for me"', 226; Reilly, 'Cleaner, carer and occasional dance partner?', 156.

32 Reilly, 'Cleaner, carer and occasional dance partner?', 156

33 Mary Copeland, in Barbara Mortimer, *Sisters: Extraordinary True-Life Stories from Nurses in World War Two* (London: Hutchinson, 2012), 227.

34 Mary Sands, 'Notes on dealing with Belsen' (April 1993), 6, MMM Belsen Concentration Camp – 1945. For some reason, Sands calls Bergen-Belsen, 'Belsen-Bergen'; it is not known why she does, but in all the documents reviewed she is the only person to refer to it in this manner.

35 K.J. Elvidge, 'Letter to "My Darling"' (26 May 1945), IWM Documents 1029.

36 Sister Penny Salter, 'Long ago and far away: A distant memory: A diary, c. 1938–1970', 157, UK Centre for the History of Nursing (hereafter UKCHN), University of Manchester; IWM Documents 17649.

37 Salter, 'Long ago and far away', 157.

38 Salter, 'Long ago and far away', 158.
39 Salter, 'Long ago and far away', 164.
40 Agnes Kathleen Dunbar Morgan, letter 58 (August 1943), CMF. 'Still with the lamp: letters to my mother by an army nursing sister. Egypt – North Africa – Sicily – Italy, 1941–1944', IWM Documents 16686.
41 Alan Gregg, 'Adaptation of survival: Reflections on our postwar problems', *American Journal of Nursing* 44, 10 (1944): 923.
42 Penny Summerfield, *Reconstructing Women's Wartime Lives: Discourse and Subjectivity in Oral Histories of the Second World War* (Manchester: Manchester University Press, 1998), 82.
43 Jessie Sarah Catherine Wilson, 'We also served, 1940 …', 61, UKCHN, University of Manchester.
44 P.M. Dyer, 'When life was grey and scarlet: A recollection of life as an Army Nursing Sister', 115–16, MMM QARANC/PE/1/151/DYER Box 8.
45 The Advisory Service of the Royal College of Nursing, 'The re-settlement of nurses'.
46 Starns, *Nurses at War*, 138.
47 Anonymous, 'Correspondence', *The British Journal of Nursing* (May 1945): 54–5.
48 'Forces obtain nurses easily', *Telegraph* (10 December 1946), Press cuttings re: nurses, MMM QARANC/PE/1/27.
49 Vera Jones, 'My dear mother and father' (29 December 1944), *A Time To Remember: A Record of Nursing Experiences, Impressions and Travels During World War II Contained in Letters Sent Home from The East* (London: Athena Press, 2005), 324. It is not known if her application was successful.
50 Anonymous, 'From all quarters'.
51 Diana Wilson, 'Obituary: Dame Monica Golding', *Independent* (25 July 1997), http://www.independent.co.uk/news/people/obituary-dame-monica-golding-1252598.html [accessed 21 October 2016].
52 For a full and detailed discussion of Margot Turner's wartime experiences and life, see John Smyth, *The Will to Live: The Story of Dame Margot Turner* (London: Hills and Lacy, 1970); Penny Starns, *Surviving Tenko: The Story of Margot Turner* (Stroud: The History Press, 2010).
53 Women, including nurses, of all allied nations were interned by the Japanese in Hong Kong, Sumatra and Malaya during the Second World War. For a detailed discussion of the lives of those women interned in Japanese camps see Lavinia Warner and John Sandilands, *Women Beyond the Wire: A Story of Prisoners of the Japanese, 1942–45* (London: Michael Joseph, 1982); Elizabeth M. Norman and Sharon Eifried, 'How did they all survive? An analysis of American nurses' experiences in Japanese Prisoner-of-War camps', *Nursing History Review* 3 (1995): 105–27; Bernice Archer and Kent Fedorowich, 'The women of Stanley: Internment in Hong Kong, 1942–45', *Women's History Review* 5, 3 (1996): 373–99;

Penny Starns, *Nurses at War: Women on the Frontline, 1939–45* (Stroud: Sutton Publishing, 2000); Christina Twomey, 'Australian nurse POWs: Gender, war and captivity', *Australian Historical Studies* 36, 124 (2004), 255–74; Christina Twomey, 'Double displacement: Western nurses return home from Japanese internment camps in Second World War', *Gender and History,* 21, 3 (2009): 670–84; Angharad Fletcher, 'Sisters behind the wire: Reappraising Australian military nursing and internment in the Pacific during World War II', *Medical History* 55 (2011): 419–24; Felicia Yap, 'Voices and silences of memory: Civilian internees of the Japanese in British Asia during the Second World War', *Journal of British Studies* 50 (2011): 917–40; Felicia Yap, 'Creativity and the body: Civilian internees in British Asia in the Second World War', in Gilly Carr and Harold Mytum (eds), *Cultural Heritage and Prisoners of War: Creativity Behind Barbed Wire* (London: Routledge, 2012); Jane Brooks, 'Wartime nursing: Feeding as forgotten practice', in Sandra B. Lewenson, Annemarie McAllister and Kylie Smith (eds), *Nursing History for Contemporary Role Development* (New York: Springer, 2017).

54 Anonymous, 'Obituaries: Brig Dame Margot Turner', MMM QARANC/RQ/2/3/2/HOVE, box 97.

55 The evidence for post-war service in the TANS by some Second World War Reservists is limited. There are no known diaries or memoirs, but medals in the medal drawers at the MMM, identify that Sister M.V.D. Hyland, Miss S.S. Epps and Cecily Earp all joined the TANS after the war ended.

56 E.R. Schofield, 'Benghazi', in Queen Alexandra's Royal Army Nursing Corps Association, *The Gazette* 3, 5 (1958): 6.

57 Anonymous, 'Eulogy: Sally Hepworth (nee Sarah Dixon)', MMM QARANC/PE/1/432/HEPW.

58 Marjorie Patricia Hunt, oral history by Conrad Wood, 10 August 1996, IWM Sound Archive 16803.

59 Katharine H. Jones, 'Miss Jane Amelia Patterson, C.B.E., R.R.C. (late Chief Principal Matron, India, QAIMNS, 1922–1947)', Queen Alexandra's Royal Army Nursing Corps Association, *The Gazette* 3, 6 (1958): 11.

60 Susan McGann, Anne Crowther and Rona Dougall, *A History of the Royal College of Nursing A Voice for Nursing, 1916–90* (Manchester: Manchester University Press, 2009), 128.

61 It is not the intention in this chapter to provide a detailed discussion on the foundation of the NHS; there is a wealth of literature on this topic. For a full and detailed account see, for example, Charles Webster, *The National Health Service: A Political History* (Oxford: Oxford University Press, 2002). For the history of nursing and the NHS see, for example, Monica E. Baly, *Nursing and Social Change* (London: Routledge, 1995); See also the special issue of the *International History of Nursing Journal*, 'Fifty years of nursing in the NHS', *International History of Nursing Journal* 3, 3 (1998).

62 Catherine Arnold Hutchinson, 'My war and welcome to it' (2001), 225. IWM Documents 11950.
63 Hutchinson, 'My war and welcome to it', 226. It appears from Hutchinson's memoir that the regime at East Grinstead was not the norm. She clearly identifies that she married and had two daughters, yet she was able to continue to work at the hospital. Hutchinson, 'My war and welcome to it', 227.
64 Anonymous, 'Covering commentary: The Second World War diaries of Miss Esther Helen Audrey Luker, ARRC', IWM Documents 1274.
65 Starns, *Nurses at War*.
66 Mortimer, *Sisters*, 294.
67 Julie Fairman and Joan E. Lynaugh, *Critical Care Nursing: A History* (Philadelphia, PA: University of Pennsylvania Press, 1998), 11.
68 Starns, *Nurses at War*, 138.
69 Starns, *Nurses at War*, 138.
70 Tyrer, *Sisters in Arms*, 303.
71 Jones, 'My dear mother and father' (30 September 1944), *A Time To Remember*, 299.
72 Bruley, *Women in Britain since 1900*, 125.
73 See, for example, Anonymous, 'Higher pay for nurses', *The Lancet* (29 December 1945): 859; Anonymous, 'New Rushcliffe Committee scales for many nursing posts', *The British Journal of Nursing* (August 1946): 90.
74 Starns, *Nurses at War*, 30. The Nurses' Salaries Committee, chaired by Lord Rushcliffe, was established in 1941 to consider nurse' salaries and conditions of work. See also McGann et al., *A History of the Royal College of Nursing*, 110–11.
75 Butland, 'Army sisters in battledress', 131. There is no information related to Butland's post-war life.
76 Anonymous, 'Editorial: For the good of all', *Nursing Times* (19 January 1946): 42.
77 Butland, 'Army sisters in battledress', 137.
78 McGann et al, *A History of the Royal College of Nursing*, 129.
79 Charles Webster, 'Nursing as the early crisis of the NHS', *International History of Nursing Journal* 3, 3 (1998): 38.
80 Anonymous, 'The grave shortage of nurses', *The British Journal of Nursing* (December 1948): 144. Nor was the problem limited to British hospitals. Sharon Richardson argues that in Canada, the shortage of recruits to hospital training programmes in the post-war era was exacerbated by the refusal of many young women to train under the harsh and hierarchical system of nurse apprenticeships. Sharon L. Richardson, '"Stand up and be counted": Nursing at the Calgary General Hospital after the Second World War', *Canadian Bulletin of Medical History* 18 (2001): 297–323.
81 Gladys B. Carter and Evelyn C. Pearce, 'The scarcity of nurses. Working conditions, domestic duties and training', *The Times* (16 May 1945), MMM

QARANC/CF/4/5/1/VARI Box 18. Gladys Carter, author of the 1939 monograph *A New Deal for Nurses*, published by Victor Gollancz, was a nurse and economist and later a member of academic staff at the Nursing Studies Unit at the University of Edinburgh. Evelyn Pearce was the senior tutor at the Middlesex Hospital School of Nursing and author of the highly influential book *A General Textbook of Nursing*, first published in 1938, which ran for at least 19 editions.

82 Gladys B. Carter, 'Reconsideration of nursing: Its fundamentals, purposes and place in the community. 3. Recruitment and training of nurses', *Nursing Mirror* (1946): 316–18.

83 Dame Katharine Jones, 'Q.A.I.M.N.S. professional and military status', *Nursing Times* (27 January 1945): 60.

84 McGann et al., *A History of the Royal College of Nursing*,135.

85 Candidus, 'The lady with the lamp is now the lady with the hump', *The Daily Sketch* (24 August 1944), MMM QARANC/CF/4/5/1/VARI Box 18.

86 For example, appointments pages in the *Nursing Times* for 7 April 1945. Several hospitals advertise for ward sisters, sister tutors and all state 'residential'. County Hospital, Dartford advertised for an assistant sister tutor: 'Salary according to service within the appropriate Rushcliffe Scale £200 to £250 a year with full residential emoluments.' Kent County Council, County Hospital, Dartford Training School for Nurses, 'Applications are invited', *Nursing Times* (7 April 1945): supplement iii; County Hospital Keighley, advertised for 'Ward sister ... Salary £130/£200 per annum together with full residential emoluments valued at £100 per annum', County Council of the West Riding of Yorkshire, County Hospital Keighley, 'Applications are invited', *Nursing Times* (7 April 1945): supplement iii; Infectious Diseases Hospital, Burnley advertised for an assistant matron, 'Rushcliffe salary, £325 to £370 per annum, less £120 value of annual emoluments', Infectious Diseases Hospital, Burnley, 'Applications are invited', *Nursing Times* (14 July 1945): supplement viii.

87 Anonymous, 'Editorial: The ward sister and professional organization', *Nursing Times* (11 August 1945): 513.

88 J. de Pinto, 'A new plan for hospital staffs', *Nursing Times* (1 December 1945): 801.

89 Anonymous, 'Editorial: Coming home – Army nurses think of demobilisation', *Nursing Times* (16 February 1946): 127.

90 Anonymous, 'Editorial: Nursing goes forward', *Nursing Times* (17 November 1945): 751. Italics in the original.

91 Anonymous, 'Editorial: For the good of all', 41–2.

92 Starns, *Nurses at War*, 150.

93 Karen Flynn, 'Proletarianization, professionalization and Caribbean immigrant nurses', *Canadian Woman Studies* 18, 1 (1998): 57–60; Julia Hallam, *Nursing the Image: Media, Culture and Professional Identity* (London:

Routledge, 2000), 121; M. Shkimba and Karen Flynn, '"In England we did nursing": Caribbean and British nurses in Great Britain and Canada, 1950–70', in Barbara Mortimer and Susan McGann (eds), *New Directions in Nursing History: International Perspectives* (London: Routledge, 2004); Diana Solano and Anne Marie Rafferty, 'Can lessons be learned from history? The origins of the British imperial nurse labour market: A discussion paper', *International Journal of Nursing Studies* 44, 6 (2007): 1055–63; McGann et al., *A History of the Royal College of Nursing*, 273–4.

94 According to Mary Sarnecky, cadet schemes in the USA were the cause of some ex-Army nurses leaving hospital nursing completely. Sarnecky, *A History of the US Army Nurse Corps*, 280.

95 Starns, *Nurses at War*, 153–4.

96 Penny Starns identifies the irony that the General Nursing Council wanted compulsory entry requirements re-introduced, and yet did not want educational reform for those candidates once they had joined the profession. Starns, *Nurses at War*, 140.

97 Hallam, *Nursing the Image*, 95.

98 David Proctor, T348, RAMC orderly and later RGN, and Arthur Brompton, T360, RAMC medic in Egypt, both RCN Oral History Archive, Edinburgh; Mortimer, *Sisters*, 299. For a useful discussion of the movement of men into nursing and the differences in how they were treated by the hospitals that employed them, see Graham J. Thurgood, 'Nurses' voices from the archives', *Journal of the Society of Archivists* 31, 2 (2010): 142.

99 McGann et al., *A History of the Royal College of Nursing*, 152.

100 One key change in the marriage rates post-war was the increase in those under 21 years of age marrying. Braybon and Summerfield suggest that whereas in 1938 one in six of all women marrying were under 21 years old, in 1945 this had increased to one in four. Gail Braybon and Penny Summerfield, *Out of the Cage: Women's Experiences in Two World Wars* (London: Pandora, 1987), 267. For a discussion on the discourse of post-war stability, see Summerfield, *Reconstructing Women's Wartime Lives*, 257–9.

101 Helen M. Sweet and Rona Dougall, *Community Nursing and Primary Healthcare in Twentieth-Century Britain* (New York: Routledge, 2008), 82.

102 I am indebted to Cyril Fish for helping with the oral history from Florence Hardy. Mrs Hardy was not able to talk herself, so Mr Fish kindly acted as an intermediary. The brief interview was taken via telephone with Mr Fish on 5 December 2013.

103 Joan Carr, oral history interview by Jane Brooks at her home in the North West, 22 November 2013, UKCHN, University of Manchester.

104 Morris, 'The diary of a wartime nurse' (23 April 1945); Morris, *A Very Private Diary* 157.

105 Ingram, 'Experiences of an Army Nurse', 10.

106 Joyce Ffoulkes Parry, *Joyce's War: The Second World War Journal of a Queen Alexandra's Imperial Military Nursing Service Nurse*, ed. Rhiannon Evans (Stroud: The History Press, 2015, Kindle edition), loc. 3604.
107 Betty Evans, oral history interview via telephone by Jane Brooks, 10 January 2014, UKCHN, University of Manchester.
108 Betty C. Parkin, *Desert Nurse: A World War II Memoir* (London: Robert Hale, 1990), 170.
109 Starns, *Nurses at War*, 138.
110 Elsie Davies, oral history interview by Jane Brooks at her home in Manchester, 18 December 2012, UKCHN, University of Manchester. Davies had not been a military nurse during the war, but having trained in Manchester from 1942 experienced war nursing as a civilian nurse. Her observations on civilian sisters are therefore particularly poignant.
111 Eileen Richardson, 'Memories of nursing', *Bulletin of the UK Association for the History of Nursing* 5 (2026): 70–2. Richardson's oral history study is based on the lives of a number of nurses who retired to the Retired Nurses' Home in Bournemouth, on the south coast of England. The home was established in the 1930s for nurses who, 'when their working time was over were unable either to find or afford accommodation for their Retirement'. Richardson, 'Memories of nursing', 70. This problem was not confined to British nurses. Lily Mary David wrote of US nurses that, 'Lack of retirement pensions and security against unemployment is the most frequent source of dissatisfaction in nursing. Rates of pay and opportunities of promotion and pay increases are also leading causes of dissatisfaction.' The most frequent reason for leaving nursing were because of marriage, but again, it is not known if fewer nurses would have left the profession for marriage if a more secure future could have been promised, or would have chosen to stay in nursing on marriage if that had been an option. Lily Mary David, 'The economic status of the nursing profession: A preliminary report of the socio-economic study, undertaken to reveal how nurses compare in their working and living conditions of women in other professions', *The American Journal of Nursing* 47, 7 (1947): 456.
112 Davies, oral history, 18 December 2012.
113 Anonymous, 'The nurse in charge', *The Lancet* (4 December 1943): 705.
114 Minister of Health, Secretary of State for Scotland and the Minister of Labour and National Service, 'Staffing the hospitals: An urgent national need', *International History of Nursing Journal* 3, 3 (1998): 15. Reprinted from pamphlet, Minister of Health, Secretary of State for Scotland and the Minister of Labour and National Service, 'Staffing the hospitals: An urgent national need' (London: HMSO, 1945) RCN Archives, Pamphlet Collection 11AD, RCN Archives, Edinburgh.
115 Richard Bessel and Dirk Schumann, 'Introduction: Violence, normality, and the construction of postwar Europe', in Richard Bessel and Dirk Schumann

(eds), *Life after Death: Approaches to a Cultural and Social History of Europe during the 1940s and 1950s* (Cambridge: Cambridge University Press, 2003).

116 In her diary of her work during the liberation of Bergen-Belsen, Sister Molly Silva Jones described her 'shame – remorse, yes, because even in 1934 we had heard of these camps and not realised, not wanted to realise that such things could happen'. Molly Silva Jones, 'From a Diary Written in Belsen', 2, IWM PP 99/86/1. See also Brooks, 'The nurse stoops down ... for me', 214.

117 For a detailed discussion of marriage, sex and child rearing in post-war Britain, see especially Pat Thane, 'Family life and "normality" in postwar British culture', in Richard Bessel and Dirk Schumann (eds), *Life after Death: Approaches to a Cultural and Social History of Europe during the 1940s and 1950s* (Cambridge: Cambridge University Press, 2003).

118 Penny Summerfield and Corinna Peniston-Bird, '"Women in the firing-line": The Home Guard and the defence of gender boundaries in Britain in the Second World War', *Women's History Review* 9, 2 (2000): 232.

119 Cynthia Enloe, *Does Khaki Become You? The Militarization of Women's Lives* (London: Pandora, 1988), 185; Summerfield, *Reconstructing Women's Wartime Lives*, 78. Summerfield pursues the narrative that women are in a no-win situation, in which they will always be expected to be two completely contradictory selves. As such, typically, they are criticised for working and not having children, and working and having children. During war this is exemplified as they are expected to work in 'men's jobs' to support the war, but not be masculine in that work and run the home too. In doing so they are unable to earn the same wage as men, their work is 'diluted', they cannot do the men's work in the same way as men, because of injunctions to be feminine and continue with domestic duties. Summerfield, *Reconstructing Women's Wartime Lives*.

120 John Costello, *Love, Sex and War: Changing Values 1939–45* (London: Collins, 1985); Enloe, *Does Khaki Become You?*, particularly 29–31; Rose, *Which People's War?*

121 Lucy Noakes, *War and the British: Gender, Memory and National Identity* (London: I.B. Tauris, 1998), 71.

122 Leisa D. Meyer, *Creating GI Jane: Sexuality and Power in the Women's Army Corps During World War II* (New York: Columbia University Press, 1996), 181.

123 This process of domesticity pervaded not only British culture. In her study of members of the Women's Army Corps, Leisa Meyer describes how one of her participants, 'was caught up in the cultural desire for normalcy and made the choice to marry shortly after discharge'. Meyer, *Creating GI Jane*, 182.

124 Arthur Salusbury MacNalty, 'Influence of war on family life', in Sir James Marchant (ed.), *Rebuilding Family Life in the Post-War World: An Enquiry with Recommendations* (London: Odhams Press, 1945), 133.

125 MacNalty, 'Influence of war on family life', 134.
126 Eliot Slater, 'Psychological aspects of family life', in Sir James Marchant (ed.), *Rebuilding Family Life in the Post-War World: An Enquiry with Recommendations* (London: Odhams Press, 1945), 100.
127 Bruley, *Women in Britain*, 125.
128 There is a significant body of literature on the position of educated professional women and students in the post-war period, all of which points to a narrowing of spheres and closing of doors. However, the picture is more complex and the return to pre-war certainties was not absolute. Carol Dyhouse argues that medical schools imposed 'quotas' on women, but they could not exclude them completely. Carol Dyhouse, 'Women students and the London medical schools, 1914–39: The anatomy of a masculine culture', *Gender and History* 10, 1 (1998): 111. Cambridge University reinstated 'quotas' for women students more generally, but from 1948 'conceded degrees' to them. Carol Dyhouse, 'Troubled identities: Gender and status in the history of the mixed college in English universities since 1945', *Women's History Review* 12, 2 (2006): 172. Girton remained an option for 'clever women', but the career choices for them on graduation were limited and about one third entered teaching. Pat Thane, 'Girton graduates: Earning and learning, 1920s–1980s', *Women's History Review* 13, 3 (2004): 354.
129 Rose, *Which People's War?*, loc. 3814.
130 Harold Smith, 'The effect of the war on the status of women', in Harold Smith (ed.), *War and Social Change: British Society in the Second World War* (Manchester: Manchester University Press, 1986), 216.
131 Noakes, *War and the British*, 72. See also Costello, *Love, Sex and War*, 370. Costello does present a more positive picture of the immediate post-war lives of young women, imagining a more permissive and open society than perhaps existed.
132 Lucy Noakes, '"Gentle in manner, resolute in deed": Women and the British army in the post-war years', *Women's History Magazine* 76 (Autumn 2014): 5; Easingwood, 'I was merely a shorthand typist'.
133 Summerfield, *Reconstructing Women's Wartime Lives*, 258.
134 Juliette Pattinson, *Behind Enemy Lines: Gender, Passing and the Special Operations Executive in the Second World War* (Manchester: Manchester University Press, 2007), 187.
135 Ali Haggart, '"Desperate housewives" and the domestic environment in post-war Britain: Individual perspectives', *Oral History* 37, 1 (2009): 53–60.
136 Summerfield, *Reconstructing Women's Wartime Lives*, 277.
137 Penny Summerfield, '"They didn't want women back in that job": The Second World War and the construction of gendered work histories', *Labour History Review* 63, 1 (1998): 84.
138 Maureen Honey, *Creating Rosie the Riveter: Class, Gender, and Propaganda*

during World War II (Amherst, MA: University of Massachusetts Press, 1984), 6.

139 The birth rate for the September quarters of the years 1941–45 was recorded as 15.7 per 1,000. In 1946 this had risen to 19.7. The rate for the September quarter of 1947 was 22 per 1,000. Figures cited from the Registrar-General's Quarterly Return of Births, Deaths and Marriages for the September Quarter (London: HMSO, 1947), cited in Anonymous, 'Central Midwives Board. The pupil's case book', *The Midwife: The British Journal of Nursing* (February 1948): 24.

140 Gail Braybon and Penny Summerfield suggest that the Treasury halved its subsidy to nurseries in 1945. Braybon and Summerfield, *Out of the Cage*, 263.

141 Deborah Montgomerie, 'Assessing Rosie: World War II, New Zealand women and the iconography of femininity', *Gender and History* 8, 1 (1996): 127.

142 Krista Cowman and Louise A. Jackson, 'Middle-class women and professional identity', *Women's History Review* 14, 2 (2005): 171.

Conclusion

From the mid-1930s, with the growing inevitability of another war, civilian nurses clamoured to join the QAs and TANS.[1] Female nurses were keen to demonstrate their skills in healing men for the war effort and to create a space for themselves as an essential part of the military medical services. The impetus for their eagerness to join the war was as much about caring for the men as it was about their personal and professional development. Sister Penny Salter wrote of the 'remarkable men I had the privilege to nurse',[2] and Sister Brenda McBryde of the tent full of 'men, reeking with blood, [which] was where I was needed'.[3] In a letter to her mother in July 1943, Sister Agnes Morgan wrote, 'Most of my love seems to be given to these men, what there is left is for you.'[4] Emma Newland's study of the civilian-made-soldier highlights the depersonalisation of the process that turned ordinary men into the machines of war.[5] *Negotiating nursing* establishes the work of nursing sisters in re-humanising these men, to support their recovery from injury and illness and remind them of why they were fighting.

This is the first book to analyse the engagement of British Army nursing sisters with their combatant patients in the Second World War. By focusing on the psychological tactics that the sisters employed in negotiating the care of their patients, it demonstrates the beginnings of a transformation of nurses from the obedient servants of the hospital to the experts by the bedside, and therefore critical to the healing of the sick. Through the examination of nursing work, this book also extends the historiography of the soldier, the critical cog in the machinery of war. The monographs of Julie Anderson and Emily Mayhew, historians of the medical war, place the soldier-patient at centre stage in a manner that this book does not.[6] Yet, although most of the personal testimonies used here come from the nurses themselves, their emphasis is invariably on the patient.

Through an uneven trajectory of developing confidence and evolving methods of patient engagement, the chapters have mapped the nurses' practices from fundamental nursing work involving body care and feeding, through the creation of homelike spaces for healing to occur, to the expansion of nursing practices into the realms of scientific medicine. In doing so, the book expands our understanding of the nature of nursing work and how medical and surgical care were successfully managed within the exigencies of limited equipment, harsh environments and inadequate medical staff. This book also honours the military nurse as a woman, often the only European woman in a war zone. It argues that far from her gender stymieing her access to the soldier-patient, it made her critical to the war effort and essential to overseas campaigns. As is argued in Chapter 3, this was not without its dangers to the nurse's professional and personal self. Furthermore, in war's wake it was their gender that forced them out of professional practice as they, along with most of their female compatriots, were encouraged back into the domestic sphere.[7]

Medical historian Mark Harrison argues that 'medicine and morale were mutually dependent', and good morale was critical for a successful military campaign.[8] The nurses, as women, 'helped to improve efficiency and boosted the morale of the patients'.[9] This dual role was not lost on the nursing sisters, who soon realised that their position on active service overseas depended upon both their clinical skills and their womanhood. However, the book argues that negotiations between gender and clinical acumen were more complex than this reductive representation of their worth. The nurses' clinical skills were a contested realm of traditional comfort care and more scientific medical roles such as the performance of anaesthesia and surgical interventions. Studies of nursing work have argued that as nurses were promoted into more senior roles, they moved away from fundamental care practices, work that was considered 'dirty', and took on more medical tasks, such as giving injections, engaging in doctors' rounds and co-ordinating care.[10] This book demonstrates that on active service overseas nursing sisters, whilst willing and excited to take on new, more scientific work, considered fundamental care to be of equal importance and critical to their vision of themselves.

Female nurses, like all women wartime workers, were caught in the interstices of conflicting roles; indeed, arguably, nurses exemplified the contradictions of women's position in war.[11] For nurses, their womanhood was fraught with paradoxes of their image as mother figures, as those with sisterly interest and as sexually knowledgeable single women with unchaperoned access to naked male bodies.[12] The incompatibility of being feminine and taking on the more scientific masculine roles required by the exigencies of active service overseas only increased the contradictions in the boundaries of nursing practice.[13] Despite the multiple anxieties surrounding the posting of female nurses into front-line areas, the needs of the soldier-patient were paramount. If the health outcomes for ill and injured combatants were improved through the intervention and presence of nursing sisters, it is also ironically the case that nurses were needed to recover them for battle and the war effort more widely.

Military success depended upon men fit to fight, and the war offered doctors the opportunity to develop their clinical skills.[14] As Anderson argues, there may be debates surrounding the benefits or otherwise of war on medicine, but there is less debate that wartime medical practice was inextricably changed by the sheer volume of those requiring treatment.[15] Cynthia Toman maintains that the Second World War was not a 'technological watershed' for nursing,[16] nor was it the professional apotheosis that some of the more celebratory texts may suggest.[17] However, as the book argues, the scale of men needing skilled nursing care and the numbers of nurses posted to active service overseas significantly revised the ways that nurses viewed their work and how they were viewed by those for whom they cared, the military authorities and their medical colleagues.[18]

There are of course limitations to this book. Whilst it has provided a comprehensive overview of the work of nursing sisters on active service overseas and examined the value that nurses and their colleagues placed on their work and participation in the war, it has not explored in detail the policy and macro-politics of their presence in war zones. By taking an original focus, specifically on personal testimony, this book has not included a quantitative analysis of British Army nurses. Of particular future interest would be studies on specific hospitals, such as the No. 1 Mobile Military Hospital, the first one of its kind to post female nurses to its contingent. A more detailed study of the work of military nurses with the female civilian inmates of Japanese POW camps would also provide additional important knowledge, as would an exploration of nurses' work with psychiatrically damaged soldier-patients. Nevertheless, despite these limitations, the value of this book lies in its examination of the manner in which nurses engaged with their patients and the innovative methods they used to salvage sick and injured men for the war effort.

Negotiating nursing has identified the problems caused when a system subordinates the female to the male. Post-war propaganda, which favoured the rights of the returning soldier to paid work, encouraged women to return to the hearth and home. As part of a female-dominated profession, nurses were not required to give up their jobs to men. However, the ideology that sent women home to care for their husbands and families meant that demobilised married nursing sisters struggled to find meaningful positions in civilian hospitals. The nation, poised as it was for the establishment of a national health service, lost some of its most talented, innovative and able nurses. Arguably, this stifled developments in practice for some years to follow.

Although the aftermath of war may have augured professional disappointment for some nursing sisters, the ramifications of the manner in which they revised nursing practice and how these evolved methods of care were understood by medical colleagues were considerable. The female nurses of the British Army had demonstrated that they could care for their patients in hostile environments, frequently under fire. They had washed soldiers, fed them, provided them with pain relief and dignity and compassion in death. The nurses had supported the sick and injured combatants' healing and given them encouragement to return to battle. Finally, on active service in the Second World War, nurses developed their practice to include scientific and highly technical work. Some of these, such as complex wound care, blood transfusions and IV therapy, were then written into the lexicon of nursing work. Other roles, such as diagnosis and prescribing, would eventually become the realm of 'advanced practice'. The contribution to nursing knowledge and practice by the nurses of the Second World War was, and remains, significant.

Notes

1 'Frontline Females', BBC Radio 4, 11 April 1998 and 18 April 1998, British Library Sound Archive H9872/2 and H9890/2.

2 Muriel Kathleen (Penny) Salter, 'Long ago and far away: A distant memory': A diary, c. 1938–1970, 29. I am indebted to Penny's friends for providing me with full access to her diary and the various press reports of her wartime nursing experiences. There is also a copy of this diary in the IWM, Documents.17649.

3 Brenda McBryde, *A Nurse's War* (Saffron Walden: Cakebread Publications, 1993), 86.

4 Agnes Kathleen Dunbar Morgan, 'My dearest mums', letter 55 (July 1943), MEF, 199, 'Still with the lamp: letters to my mother by an army nursing sister. Egypt – North Africa – Sicily – Italy, 1941–1944', IWM Documents 16686.

5 Emma Newlands, *Civilians into Soldiers: War, the Body and British Army Recruits, 1939–45* (Manchester: Manchester University Press, 2014).

6 Emily Mayhew, *The Reconstruction of Warriors: Archibald McIndoe, The Royal Air Force and the Guinea Pig Club* (Barnsley: Greenhill Books, Kindle edition, 2010); Julie Anderson, *War, Disability and Rehabilitation in Britain: 'Soul of a Nation'* (Manchester: Manchester University Press, 2011).

7 Most literature on women's work in the Second World War offers analyses of the post-war return to the home and hearth. See, for example, Gail Braybon and Penny Summerfield, *Out of the Cage: Women's Experiences in Two World Wars* (London: Pandora, 1987); Sonya O. Rose, *Which People's War? National Identity and Citizenship in Britain, 1939–1945* (Oxford: Oxford University Press, 2003); Lucy Noakes, *Women in the British Army: War and the Gentle Sex, 1907–1948* (London: Routledge, Kindle edition, 2006).

8 Mark Harrison, *Medicine and Victory: British Military Medicine in the Second World War* (Oxford: Oxford University Press, 2004), 199.

9 Harrison, *Medicine and Victory*, 219.

10 See the testimony of Lisbeth Hockey, 'People don't perceive hands-on nursing as being skilled nursing. The minute you gave them an injection … I think your reputation rose.' Barbara Mortimer, *Sisters: Extraordinary True-Life Stories from Nurses in World War Two* (London: Hutchinson, 2012), 130. See also Jocalyn Lawler, *Behind the Screens: Nursing, Somology and the Problem of the Body* (Melbourne: Churchill Livingstone, 1991). For a useful discussion of the increase in professional prestige as nurses move away from the bedside, see Jean McIntosh and Robert Dingwall's analysis of the relationship between nursing and health visiting. Jean McIntosh and Robert Dingwall, 'Teamwork in theory and practice', in Robert Dingwall and Jean McIntosh (eds), *Readings in the Sociology of Nursing* (Edinburgh: Churchill Livingstone, 1978).

11 Penny Summerfield, *Reconstructing Women's Wartime Lives: Discourse*

and Subjectivity in Oral Histories of the Second World War (Manchester: Manchester University Press, 1998), 24; Penny Summerfield and Corinna Peniston-Bird, 'Women in the firing-line: The Home Guard and the defence of gender boundaries in Britain in the Second World War', *Women's History Review* 9, 2 (2000): 232.

12 Noakes, *Women in the British Army*, 127.

13 For a useful and erudite examination of the involvement of nurses in science and technology, see, for example, Julie Fairman and Patricia D'Antonio, 'Virtual power: Gendering the nurse–technology relationship', *Nursing Inquiry* 6, 3 (1999): 178–86.

14 Newlands, *Civilians into Soldiers.*

15 Anderson, *War, Disability and Rehabilitation in Britain*, 74.

16 Cynthia Toman, *An Officer and a Lady: Canadian Military Nursing and the Second World War* (Vancouver: University of British Columbia Press, 2007), 201.

17 See, for example, Juliet Piggott, *Queen Alexandra's Royal Army Nursing Corps* (London, Leo Cooper, 1975); Eric Taylor, *Women Who Went to War, 1938–46* (London: Robert Hale, 1988); Eric Taylor, *Front-Line Nurse: British Nurses in World War II* (London: Robert Hale, 1997); Eric Taylor, *Combat Nurse* (London: Robert Hale, 1999); Eric Taylor, *Wartime Nurse: 100 years from the Crimea to Korea 1854–1954* (London: Robert Hale, 2001).

18 Toman, *An Officer and a Lady*, 10. F.A.E. Crew, 'The Army medical services', in Arthur Salusbury MacNalty and W. Franklin Mellor (eds), *Medical Services in War: The Principal Medical Lessons of the Second World War* (London: HMSO, 1968), 77–81. There are numerous examples of the impact that individual nursing sisters had on their patients' recovery and the developing collegiality between nursing sisters and medical officers. For a range of these, see, for example, the testimonies of Sister Sheena Kilminster, Ward Sister Isobel Balmain and Sister Monica Baly in Mortimer, *Sisters*, 190–1, 193–4, 200.

Bibliography

Archives

British Library
Imperial War Museum
Museum of Military Medicine (formerly Army Medical Museum)
The National Archives, Kew
Princess Mary's Royal Air Force Nursing Service Archive
Royal College of Nursing Archive, Edinburgh
Wellcome Library, London

Oral histories

(Unless otherwise stated all oral histories are held at the UK Centre for the History of Nursing, at the University of Manchester)

Bowring, Elizabeth, oral history interview via telephone by Jane Brooks, 31 July 2012

Carr, Joan, oral history interview by Jane Brooks, at her home in the north-west of England, 22 November 2013.

Cash, Marion, oral history interview via telephone by Jane Brooks, 23 October 2013.

Cheetham, John, oral history interview by Jane Brooks, at his home in the north-west of England, 8 September 2012.

Christie, Cecelia Helen Burnette, oral history interview by Conrad Wood, 25 March 1993, IWM Sound Archive, 13121

Clarke, Jean, oral history interview via telephone by Jane Brooks, 20 November 2013.

Cooper, Gertrude Annie, oral history interview by Margaret Skellern, 10 May 1994. Royal College of Nursing Oral History Archive, Edinburgh.

Cottrell, Evelyn Alma, Spears Unit, oral history interview by Lyn E. Smith, 9 July 1990, IWM Oral History Collection, Interview 12180.

Crisp, Betty, oral history interview via telephone by Jane Brooks, 13 January 2014.

Davies, Elsie, oral history interview by Jane Brooks at her home in Manchester, 18 December 2012.

Dowling, Ursula, oral history interview by Rosemary Hart on behalf of the BBC, 1986, IWM Oral History Collection, Interview 9910.

Dunnett, Amy Selina (Pam), oral history interview by Lyn E. Smith, 25 March 1999, IWM Sound Archive, 18784.

Edwards, Jean, oral history interview via telephone by Jane Brooks, 6 November 2013.

Evans, Betty, oral history interview via telephone by Jane Brooks, 10 January 2014.

'Frontline Females', BBC Radio 4, 11 April 1998 and 18 April 1998: British Library Sound Archive H9872/2 and H9890/2. In this programme Claire Rayner discussed their wartime nursing experiences with Monica Baly, Mary Bates, Glenys Branson, Constance Collingwood, Gertrude Cooper, Ursula Dowling, Brenda Fuller, Anne Gallimore, Monica Goulding, Daphne Ingram, Anita Kelly, Margaret Kneebone, Sylvia Mayo, Kay McCormack, Anne Moat, Phyllis Thoms and Margot Turner.

Haddie Swan, Mary, oral history interview by Lyn E. Smith, 26 October 1998, IWM Sound Archive, 18571.

Hamilton, June (pseudonym) oral history interview by Jane Brooks at her home in the south of England, 19 October 2011.

Hardy, Florence, born in 1916 and trained in London. Given Mrs Hardy's age it was not possible to interview her in person, but I liaised with her via her great friend Mr Cyril Fish via telephone, 5 December 2013.

Morris, Elizabeth, oral history interview via telephone by Jane Brooks, 8 October 2013.

Newton, Bessie, oral history interview by Jane Brooks, at her home in Yorkshire, 21 April 2012.

Nicolson, Joan Eileen, oral history by Conrad Wood, 8 June 1991, IWM Sound Archive 12075.

Parkes, Margaret, oral history interview by Jane Brooks at her home in the north-west of England, 12 December 2012.

Peake, Joan (nee Botting), oral history by her son, Andrew Peake, 17 March 1993, Royal College of Nursing Oral History Archive, Edinburgh.

Potter, Evelyn (pseudonym), oral history interview via telephone by Jane Brooks, 16 September 2013.

Slater, Rachel (pseudonym), oral history interview by Jane Brooks in the south of England, 20 October 2011.

Soper, Emily, oral history interview via the telephone by Jane Brooks, 6 September 2013.

Personal testimonies

(Unless otherwise stated all personal testimonies are held at the UK Centre for the History of Nursing, at the University of Manchester)

Baker, C.M.S., 'Aftermath of war, September 1945' and 'A view of war by an officer of the QAIMNS, October 1943 to May 1945', Imperial War Museum Private Papers (hereafter IWM) Documents 6341.
Bower, Iris, OBE, ARRC, 'From Normandy to the Baltic' (October 1985).
Briggs, Phyllis Mary, 'Alor Star', IWM Documents 4419.
Brown, Francie E., letters to Mrs W.R. Trotman (10 September 1942–4 August 1944), IWM Documents 12472.
Butland, Catherine M., 'Army sisters in battledress or the chosen few or follow fate', MMM, QARANC/PE/1/74/BUTL Box 8.
Collins, Barbara, 'Letters home from Sierra Leone', 1940–1941.
Dyer, P.M., 'When life was grey and scarlet: A recollection of life as an Army Nursing Sister', MMM, QARANC/PE/1/151/DYER Box 8.
Elvidge, Kathleen J., 'Letter to "My Darling"' (26 May 1945), IWM Documents 1029.
Feggetter, George, 'Diary of an R.A.M.C. surgeon at war, 1942–1946', Wellcome Library, London, RAMC 1776.
Hutchinson, Catherine Arnold, 'My war and welcome to it' (2001), IWM Documents 11950.
Ingram, Daphne (nee de Wart), 'Experiences of an army nurse: POW with Japanese', IWM Documents 2319.
Jarrett, Nell, 'Diary of her desert experiences' (21 June 1942–13 January 1943).
Leeming, E.M., 'My war years, 1939–1945', Wellcome Library, London, PP/LEE.
Luker, Esther Helen Audrey, ARRC, 'Diaries from 1940–45', IWM Documents 1274.
McDonald, J.R., 'A doctor goes to war', Wellcome Library London, RAMC 944.
Morgan, Agnes Kathleen Dunbar, 'Still with the lamp: Letters to my mother by an army nursing sister. Egypt – North Africa – Sicily – Italy, 1941–1944', IWM Documents 16686.
Morris, Mary, 'The diary of a wartime nurse', IWM Documents 4850.
Mountford, Winifred Margaret (later Winstanley), 'Monty', unpublished memoir of her wartime experiences as a QAIMNS Sister in the Second World War.
Radloff, Ann, 'Going to Gooseberry Beach: Travels and adventures of a nursing sister', IWM Documents.147.
Salter, Muriel Kathleen (Penny), 'Long ago and far away: A distant memory': A diary, c. 1938–1970. There is also a copy of this diary in the IWM, Documents 17649.
Silva Jones, Molly, 'From a diary written in Belsen', IWM Documents 9550.

Stevenson, Edith, 'The last lap: Autobiography 1912–1986', 3. IWM LBY 94 / 1636.
Wilson, Sister Jessie Sarah Catherine, 'We also served, 1940 …'.

Government and professional reports

The Advisory Service of the Royal College of Nursing, 'The re-settlement of nurses: Back to civilian life' (London: H. and Co., December 1945).
The Lancet Commission on Nursing, *Final Report* (London: The Lancet, 1932).
Ministry of Health, Board of Education and Department of Health for Scotland (Chairman, Earl of Athlone), *Interim Report of the Inter-Departmental Committee on Nursing Services* (London: HMSO, 1939).
Ministry of Health, *First Report of Nurses' Salaries Committee* (London: HMSO, 1943).

Published primary sources

Anonymous, 'The technique of blood transfusion', *Nursing Mirror* (2 September 1939): 764.
Anonymous, 'War – what it means to the nurse', *Nursing Mirror and Midwives' Journal* (2 September 1939): 755.
Anonymous, 'Editorial: Tannic acid "is out"', *Nursing Mirror and Midwives' Journal* (23 November 1940): 171.
Anonymous, 'Editorial: War-time advances and antiseptics', *Nursing Times* (11 April 1942): 237.
Anonymous, 'Nursing adventure: The story of two nursing sisters returning on the torpedoed "*Rangitane*"', *Nursing Times* (25 October 1942): 672.
Anonymous, 'Penicillin saves wounded soldiers', *The British Journal of Nursing* (September 1943):104.
Anonymous, 'The nurse in charge', *The Lancet* (4 December 1943): 705.
Anonymous, 'Penicillin in the field', *The Lancet* (11 December 1943): 737.
Anonymous, 'News from the nursing world: Professor Florey on penicillin', *Nursing Mirror and Midwives' Journal* (18 December 1943): 161.
Anonymous, 'Penicillin in the treatment of war wounds', *Nursing Times* (8 January 1944): 19.
Anonymous, 'Editorial: Penicillin treatment reviewed', *Nursing Times* (22 April 1944): 275.
Anonymous, 'Topical notes – Normandy broadcast', *Nursing Times* (1 July 1944): 430.
Anonymous, 'In Step with the QAs 1. – An officer writes to his wife from the Anzio beachhead', *Nursing Times* (5 August 1944): 538.
Anonymous, 'In step with the QAs 8. – Hospital ship (Part I)', *Nursing Times* (30 September 1944): 678.

Anonymous, 'In step with the QAs 9. – Hospital ship (part II)', *Nursing Times* (7 October 1944): 698.
Anonymous, 'Penicillin for P.O.W.', *British Medical Journal* (7 October 1944): 484.
Anonymous, 'Penicillin: Indications for its use and methods of administration', *Nursing Mirror* (14 April 1945): 16.
Anonymous, 'Penicillin: Indications for its use and methods of administration', *The British Journal of Nursing* (April 1945): 39.
Anonymous, 'Correspondence', *The British Journal of Nursing* (May 1945): 54–55.
Anonymous, 'Editorial: The ward sister and professional organization', *Nursing Times* (11 August 1945): 513.
Anonymous, 'Editorial: Nursing goes forward', *Nursing Times* (17 November 1945): 751.
Anonymous, 'Higher pay for nurses', *The Lancet* (29 December 1945): 859.
Anonymous, 'Editorial: For the good of all', *Nursing Times* (19 January 1946): 41–42.
Anonymous, 'Coming home – Army nurses think of demobilisation', *Nursing Times* (16 February 1946): 127.
Anonymous, 'Living out and living in', *Nursing Mirror* (2 March 1946): 361–2.
Anonymous, 'New Rushcliffe Committee scales for many nursing posts', *The British Journal of Nursing* (August 1946): 90.
Anonymous, 'Central Midwives Board. The pupil's case book', *The Midwife: The British Journal of Nursing* (February 1948): 24.
Anonymous, 'The grave shortage of nurses', *The British Journal of Nursing* (December 1948): 144.
B.B., Sister, 'Nursing in Belsen Camp', *Nursing Times* (14 July 1945): 204.
Barford, A.M., 'Nurse anaesthetics', *British Medical Journal* (5 October 1940): 474.
Bartlett, Dorothy A., *Nurse in War* (London: P.R. Macmillan, 1961).
Beardwell, Myrtle, *Aftermath* (Ilfracombe: Arthur Stockwell, c. 1953).
Bevington, Sheila M., *Nursing Life and Discipline: A Study Based on Over Five Hundred Interviews* (London: H.K. Lewis, 1943).
Bolton, Angela, *The Maturing Sun: An Army Nurse in India 1942–45* (London: Headline, 1986).
Bond, Mary, *Wartime Experiences from the Midnight Sun to Belsen* (Cardigan: E.L. Jones and Son, 1994).
Bowden, Jean, *Grey Touched with Scarlet: The War Experiences of Army Nursing Sisters* (London: Robert Hale, 1959).
Bright, Pamela, *Life in our Hands: Nursing Sister's War Experiences* (London: Pan Books, 1955).
Bunyan, John, 'Treatment of wounds and burns by the envelope method', *Nursing Times* 72 (22 February 1941): supplement, ii–iii.

Carter, Gladys B., 'Reconsideration of nursing: Its fundamentals, purposes and place in the community. 3. Recruitment and training of nurses', *Nursing Mirror* (1946): 316–18.

Dale, H.E., 'Modern drugs: 3 – Penicillin', *Nursing Times* (27 November 1943): 883.

Darley, V.E., 'Living out is *not* such an advantage', *Nursing Mirror* (23 March 1946): 424.

David, Lily Mary, 'The economic status of the nursing profession: A preliminary report of the socio-economic study, undertaken to reveal how nurses compare in their working and living conditions of women in other professions', *The American Journal of Nursing* 47, 7 (1947): 456–62.

de Pinto, J., 'A new plan for hospital staffs', *Nursing Times* (1 December 1945): 801.

Dick, Bruce M., 'Injuries and wounds of the chest', in J.M. Mackintosh, *Wartime Nurse: An Anthology of Ideas about the Care and Nursing of War Casualties* (Edinburgh: Oliver and Boyd, 1940).

Dickens, Monica, *Chronicle of a Working Life: One Pair of Feet* (Stroud: Sutton Publishing, 2004).

Edge, Geraldine, and Johnston, Mary E., *Ships of Youth: The Experiences of Two Army Nursing Sisters on Board the Hospital Carrier Leinster* (London: Hodder and Stoughton, 1945).

Elam, John, 'Anaesthesia in war-time', *The Lancet* (15 April 1939): 906.

Elam, John, 'Nurse anaesthetists', *The British Medical Journal* (14 September 1940): 368.

Emergency Medical Services, Ministry of Health, 'Memorandum: The treatment of burns', *Nursing Times* (5 April 1941): 242.

Fletcher, C.M., 'Penicillin: A recent advance in chemotherapy', *Nursing Times* (4 October 1941): 798–800.

Goode, Alan F., 'Correspondence', *British Medical Journal* (28 September 1940): 430.

Gordon, J. Elsie, 'With the BAFO and BAOR – 4: In the depressing city of Berlin', *Nursing Times* (8 December 1945): 157–8.

Gregg, Alan, 'Adaptation of survival: Reflections on our postwar problems', *American Journal of Nursing* 44, 10 (1944): 923.

Harries, E.H.R, Swyer, Robert, and Thompson, Noel, 'Sulphanilamide in typhoid fever', *The Lancet* (10 June 1939): 1321–4.

Harrison, Ada (ed.), *Grey and Scarlet: Letters from the War Areas by Army Sisters on Active Service* (London: Hodder and Stoughton, 1944).

Henderson, R.G., 'Treatment of incendiary bomb burns', *Nursing Mirror* (6 July 1940): 325–6.

Hilder, Joyce C., 'All in the day's work IV.– Darkest Africa!', *Nursing Times* 38, 1919 (7 February 1942): 93.

I.B.H., 'In step with the QAs 2. – Nursing in a psychiatric hospital for officers', *Nursing Times* (12 August 1944): 557.

Jones, Dame Katharine, 'On active service with the Army', *Nursing Times* (25 September 1943): 719–20.

Jones, Dame Katharine, 'Broadcast talk to North America', *The British Journal of Nursing* (November 1943): 124–5.

Jones, Dame Katharine, 'QAIMNS professional and military status', *Nursing Times* (27 January 1945): 60–1, 67.

Jones, Katharine H., 'Introduction', in Ada Harrison (ed.), *Grey and Scarlet: Letters from the War Areas by Army Sisters on Active Service* (London: Hodder and Stoughton, 1944).

Jones, Katharine H., 'Miss Jane Amelia Patterson, CBE, RRC (late Chief Principal Matron, India, QAIMNS, 1922–1947)', in Queen Alexandra's Royal Army Nursing Corps Association, *The Gazette* 3, 6 (1958): 11.

Jones, Vera, *A Time To Remember: A Record of Nursing Experiences, Impressions and Travels during World War II Contained in Letters Sent Home from the East* (London: Athena Press, 2005).

K.M.C., 'In step with the QAs 6'. – Blitz on George Cross Island', *Nursing Times* (16 September 1944): 643–4.

La Motte, Ellen Newbold, *The Backwash of War: The Human Wreckage of the Battlefield as Witnessed by an American Hospital Nurse* (New York: G.P. Putnam's Sons, 2016).

Layton, T.B., 'Transport of wounded: Surgical aspects', *The Lancet* (23 March 1940): 537–40.

Learmonth, J.R., 'The surgical nurse', in J.M. Mackintosh, *Wartime Nurse: An Anthology of Ideas about the Care and Nursing of War Casualties* (Edinburgh: Oliver and Boyd, 1940).

Lipscombe, F.M., 'Medical aspects of Belsen concentration camp', *The Lancet* (8 September 1945): 313–15.

Logie, N.J., 'Treatment of burns in Tobruk', *Nursing Mirror* (10 July 1943): 230.

Love Tayloe, Roberta, *Combat Nurse: A Journal of World War II* (Santa Barbara, CA: Fithian Press, 1988).

McAdam, I.W.J., Duguid, J.P., and Challinor, S.W., 'Systemic administration of penicillin', *The Lancet* (9 September 1944): 336.

McBryde, Brenda, *A Nurse's War* (Saffron Walden: Cakebread Publications, 1993).

MacCormick, Iain, *The Feminine Touch.* Director, Pat Jackson (27 March 1956), Ealing Studios, www.imdb.com/title/tt0050428/ [accessed 28 September 2016].

McIndoe, Archibald H., 'Saline baths treatment for burns', *Nursing Mirror* (18 July 1942): i–ii.

Mackintosh, J.M., *Wartime Nurse: An Anthology of Ideas about the Care and Nursing of War Casualties* (Edinburgh: Oliver and Boyd, 1940).

MacNalty, Arthur Salusbury, 'Influence of war on family life', in Sir James Marchant (ed.), *Rebuilding Family Life in the Post-War World: An Enquiry with Recommendations* (London: Odhams Press, 1945).

Mitchiner, Philip, 'Modern methods of treating war burns', *Nursing Mirror* (10 May 1943): 23–4.
Moody, Patricia, 'With pen and brush – a QA reports. 3. – When a ward is a tent', *Nursing Times* (25 November 1944): 810.
Moody, Patricia, 'With pen and brush – a QA reports. 4. – Night duty – with a difference', *Nursing Times* 40 (2 December 1944): 829.
Morris, Mary, *A Very Private Diary: A Nurse in Wartime*, ed. Carol Acton (London: Weidenfeld and Nicolson, 2014).
Murphy, J.D.F., 'The insulin coma unit in a military psychiatric division', *Journal of the Royal Army Medical Corps* 99 (1953): 232–43.
Nicol, A.A., *My Moving Tent: Diary of a Desert Rat* (Edinburgh: Pentland Press, 1994).
Nightingale, Florence, 'Subsidiary note as to the introduction of female nursing into military hospitals in peace and in war' (Thoughts submitted as to an eventual Nurses' Provident Fund), Presented to the Secretary of State for War (London: Harrison and Son, 1858).
Nightingale, Florence, *Notes on Nursing: What It Is and What It Is Not* (New York: Dover Publications, 1969).
Park, R.G., 'Cutaneous hypersensitivity to sulphonamides: A report of 12 cases', *The British Medical Journal* 2, 4306 (17 July 1943): 69–72.
Parkin, Betty C., *Desert Nurse: A World War II Memoir* (London: Robert Hale, 1990).
Parsons, F.B., 'Nurse anaesthetists', *British Medical Journal* (28 September 1940): 429.
Pearce, Evelyn, *A General Textbook of Nursing: A Comprehensive Guide to the Final State Examinations* (London: Faber and Faber, 1937).
Philip, Cornelius B., 'Tsutsugamushi disease (scrub typhus) in World War II', *The Journal of Parasitology* 34, 3 (June 1948): 169–91.
Romanis, W.H.C., 'Amputation in war time', *Nursing Times* (15 June 1940): 266–7.
Schofield, E.R., 'Benghazi', in Queen Alexandra's Royal Army Nursing Corps Association, *The Gazette* 3, 5 (1958): 5–7.
Skimming, Sylvia, *Sand in My Shoes: The Tale of a Red Cross Welfare Officer with British Hospitals Overseas in the Second World War* (Edinburgh: Oliver and Boyd, 1948).
Slater, Eliot, 'Psychological aspects of family life', in Sir James Marchant (ed.), *Rebuilding Family Life in the Post-War World: An Enquiry with Recommendations* (London: Odhams Press, 1945).
Stanford Read, Charles, 'The nurse and the psychological emergencies of war', *Nursing Mirror* (16 September 1939): 319–20.
Stanley-Sykes, W., 'Nurse anaesthetists', *British Medical Journal* (1 March 1941): 339.
Stokes, John F., 'The present status of the sulphonamide drugs', *Nursing Times* (21 February 1942): 124–5.

Telshaw Camp, LaVonne, *Lingering Fever: A World War II Nurse's Memoir* (Jefferson, NC: McFarland, 1997).
Turner, S.C., 'All in the day's work. III – Nursing on a troopship', *Nursing Times* (17 January 1942): 76.
Wakeley, Cecil P.G,. 'The treatment of war burns', *Nursing Times* (11 October 1941): 819–24.
Weeks-Shaw, Clara, *A Text-Book of Nursing: For the Use of Training Schools, Families and Private Students* (3rd edn) (New York: D. Appleton and Company, 1906).
Wells, C.A., 'Post-war pattern: War-time advances in surgery', *Nursing Times* (9 June 1945): 368–69 and 373.
Wilks, Janet, *Carbolic and Leeches* (Ilfracombe: Arthur H. Stockwell, 1991).
Woods, H.B., 'Treatment of severe war-time burns', *Nursing Times* (5 November 1943): 821, 827 and 833.

Secondary sources

Abrams, Lynn, *Oral History Theory* (London: Routledge, 2010).
Abrams, Lynn, 'Liberating the female self: Epiphanies, conflict and coherence in the life stories of post-war British women', *Social History* 39, 1 (2014): 14–35.
Acton, Carol, '"Stepping into history": Reading the Second World War through Irish women's diaries', *Irish Studies Review* 18, 1 (2010): 39–56.
Adams, Iain, 'A game for Christmas? The Argylls, Saxons and football on the Western Front, December 1914', *The International Journal of the History of Sport* 32, 11–12 (2015): 1395–415.
Aiston, Sarah, 'A maternal identity? The family lives of British women graduates pre- and post-1945', *History of Education* 34, 4 (2005): 407–26.
Alwis, Anne P., 'Men in pain: masculinity, medicine and the *Miracles* of St. Artemios', *Byzantine and Modern Greek Studies* 36, 1 (2012): 1–19.
Anderson, Julie, *War, Disability and Rehabilitation in Britain: 'Soul of a Nation'* (Manchester: Manchester University Press, 2011).
Archer, Bernice, and Fedorowich, Kent, 'The women of Stanley: Internment in Hong Kong, 1942–45', *Women's History Review* 5, 3 (1996): 373–99.
Astedt-Kurki, Paivi, and Isola, Arja, 'Humour between nurses and patient, and among staff: Analysis of nurses' diaries', *Journal of Advanced Nursing* 35, 3 (2001): 452–8.
Baly, Monica E., *Nursing and Social Change* (London: Routledge, 1995).
Bardgett, Suzanne, and Cesarani, David (eds), *Belsen 1945, New Historical Perspectives* (London: Vallentine Mitchell, 2006).
Bashford, Alison, *Purity and Pollution: Gender, Embodiment and Victorian Medicine* (Basingstoke: Macmillan, 1998).
Bassett, Jan, *Guns and Brooches: Australian Army Nursing from the Boer War to the Gulf War* (Oxford: Oxford University Press, 1992).

Beaumont, Caitriona, 'Citizens not feminists: The boundary negotiated between citizenship and feminism by mainstream women's organisations in England, 1928–39', *Women's History Review* 9, 2 (2000): 411–29.

Beaumont, Caitriona, 'The women's movement, politics and citizenship, 1918–1950s', in Ina Zweiniger-Bargielowska (ed.), *Women in Twentieth-Century Britain* (Harlow: Pearson Education, 2001).

Beck, Cheryl Tatano, 'Humor in nursing practice: A phenomenological study', *International Journal of Nursing Studies* 34, 5 (1997): 346–52.

Benjamin, David, 'Afterword', *The Home: Words, Interpretations, Meanings and Environments* (Aldershot: Ashgate, 1995).

Berger Gluck, Sherna, and Patai, Daphne, 'Introduction', in Sherna Berger Gluck and Daphne Patai (eds), *Women's Words: The Feminist Practice of Oral History* (London: Routledge, 1991).

Bessel, Richard, and Schumann, Dirk (eds), *Life after Death: Approaches to a Cultural and Social History of Europe during the 1940s and 1950s* (Cambridge: Cambridge University Press, 2003).

Bessel, Richard, and Schumann, Dirk, 'Introduction: Violence, normality, and the construction of postwar Europe', in Richard Bessel and Dirk Schumann (eds), *Life after Death: Approaches to a Cultural and Social History of Europe during the 1940s and 1950s* (Cambridge: Cambridge University Press, 2003).

Biedermann, Narelle, 'The voices of days gone by: Advocating the use of oral history in nursing', *Nursing Inquiry* 8 (2001): 61–2.

Bingham, Adrian, '"An era of domesticity": Histories of women and gender in interwar Britain', *Cultural and Social History* 1 (2004): 225–33.

Bingham, Adrian, 'Enfranchisement, feminism and the modern woman: Debates in the British popular press, 1918–1939', in Julie V. Gottlieb and Richard Toye (eds), *The Aftermath of Suffrage: Women, Gender, and Politics in Britain 1918–1945* (Basingstoke: Palgrave Macmillan, 2013).

Bland, Lucy, 'White women and men of colour: Miscegenation fears in Britain after the Great War', *Gender and History* 17, 1 (2005): 29–61.

Bornat, Joanna, 'A second take: Revisiting interviews with a different purpose', *Oral History* 31, 1 (2003): 47–53.

Boschma, Geertje, Scaia, Margaret, Bonifacio, Nerrisa, and Roberts, Erica, 'Oral history research', in Sandra B. Lewenson and Eleanor Krohn Herrmann (eds), *Capturing Nursing History: A Guide to Historical Methods in Research* (New York: Springer, 2008).

Boschma, Geertje, Roberts, Erica, Dhari, Ranjit, Mahabir, Gilda, Walter, Susan, and Haney, Catherine, '"Nobody ever asked me about my career": Public health nurses' oral histories preserved', *The Bulletin of the UK Association for the History of Nursing* 4 (2015): 43–51.

Bourke, Joanna, *Dismembering the Male: Men's Bodies, Britain and the Great War* (London: Reaktion Books, 1996).

Bourke, Joanna, 'Disciplining the emotions: Fear, psychiatry and the Second

World War', in Roger Cooter, Mark Harrison and Steve Sturdy (eds), *War, Medicine and Modernity* (Stroud: Sutton Publishing, 1998).

Bourke, Joanna, *The Second World War: A People's History* (Oxford: Oxford University Press, 2001).

Bourke, Joanna, *The Story of Pain: From Prayer to Painkillers* (Oxford: Oxford University Press, 2014).

Braybon, Gail, and Summerfield, Penny, *Out of the Cage: Women's Experiences in Two World Wars* (London: Pandora, 1987).

Brock, Julia, Dickey, Jennifer W., Harker, Richard J.W., and Lewis, Catherine M. (eds), *Beyond Rosie: A Documentary History of Women and World War II* (Fayetteville, AK: University of Arkansas Press, 2015, Kindle edition).

Brooks, Jane, '"Visiting rights only": The early experience of nurses in higher education, 1918–1960' [unpublished PhD thesis] (London: London School of Hygiene and Tropical Medicine, 2005).

Brooks, Jane, '"Uninterested in anything except food": Nurse feeding work with the liberated inmates of Bergen-Belsen', *Journal of Clinical Nursing* 21 (2012): 2958–65.

Brooks, Jane, 'Nursing typhus victims in the Second World War, 1942–1944', *Journal of Advanced Nursing* 70, 7 (2014): 1510–19.

Brooks, Jane, '"The nurse stoops down ... for me": Nursing the liberated persons at Bergen-Belsen', in Jane Brooks and Christine E. Hallett (eds), *One Hundred Years of Nursing Wartime Practices, 1854–1953* (Manchester: Manchester University Press, 2015).

Brooks, Jane, 'Wartime nursing: Feeding as forgotten practice', in Sandra B. Lewenson, Annemarie McAllister and Kylie Smith (eds), *Nursing History for Contemporary Role Development* (New York: Springer, 2017).

Brooks, Jane, and Hallett, Christine E., 'Introduction: The practice of nursing and the exigencies of war', in Jane Brooks and Christine E. Hallett (eds), *One Hundred Years of Wartime Nursing Practices, 1854–1953* (Manchester: Manchester University Press, 2015).

Brooks, Jane, and Hallett, Christine E. (eds), *One Hundred Years of Nursing Wartime Practices, 1854-1953* (Manchester: Manchester University Press, 2015).

Brooks, Jane, and Rafferty, Anne Marie, 'Dress and distinction in nursing, 1860–1945: "A corporate (as well as corporeal) armour of probity and purity"', *Women's History Review* 16, 1 (2007): 41–57.

Brown, Kevin, *Fighting Fit: Health, Medicine and War in the Twentieth Century* (Stroud: The History Press, 2008, Kindle edition).

Brown, William R., 'The American girl and the Christmas tree: World War II soldier poets look at what the GIs were fighting for', *Journal of American Culture* 8, 2 (1985): 25–30.

Bruley, Sue, *Women in Britain since 1900* (Basingstoke: Palgrave Macmillan, 1999).

Brundage, Anthony, *Going to the Sources: A Guide to Historical Research and Writing* (Hoboken, NJ: Wiley Blackwell, 2017).

Bud, Robert, *Penicillin: Triumph and Tragedy* (Oxford: Oxford University Press, 2007).

Buhler-Wilkerson, Karen, *No Place Like Home: A History of Nursing and Home Care in the United States* (Baltimore, MD: Johns Hopkins University Press, 2001).

Burke Odland, Sarah, 'Unassailable Motherhood, Ambivalent Domesticity: The Construction of Maternal Identity in Ladies' Home Journal in 1946', *Journal of Communication Inquiry* 34, 1 (2010): 61–84.

Burris, Marsha L., *Paradox of Professionalism: American Nurses in World War II* (Charlotte: Spiral Publications, 2007).

Byrski, Liz, 'Emotional labour as war work: Women up close and personal with McIndoe's Guinea Pigs', *Women's History Review* 21, 3 (July 2012): 341–61.

Cade, Stanford, 'Burns in the Royal Air Force', *Medical Training Establishment and Dept Royal Air Force Journal* 1 (1941): 1–2.

Caine, Barbara, *English Feminism, 1780–1980* (Oxford: Oxford University Press, 2001).

Callaway, Barbara J., *Hildegard Peplau: Psychiatric Nurse of the Century* (New York: Springer, 2002).

Canning, Deebs, Rosenberg, John P., and Yates, Patsy, 'Therapeutic relationships in specialist palliative care nursing practice', *International Journal of Palliative Nursing* 13, 5 (2007): 222–9.

Canning, Kathleen, 'The body as method? Reflections on the place of the body in gender history', *Gender and History* 11, 3 (1999): 499–513.

Carden-Coyne, Ana, *The Politics of Wounds: Military Patients and Medical Power in the First World War* (Oxford: Oxford University Press, 2014).

Carr, Gilly, and Mytum, Harold (eds), *Cultural Heritage and Prisoners of War: Creativity Behind Barbed Wire* (London: Routledge, 2012)

Carr, Gilly, Sanders, Paul, and Willmot, Louise (eds), *Protest, Defiance and Resistance in the Channel Islands German Occupation, 1940–45* (London: Bloomsbury, 2014).

Celinscak, Mark, 'At war's end: Allied forces at Bergen-Belsen' [unpublished PhD thesis] (Toronto: York University, 2012).

Church, Olga M., and Johnson, M.L., 'Worth remembering: The process and products of oral history', *International History of Nursing Journal* 1, 1 (1995): 23–4.

Connerton, Winifred, 'American nurses in colonial settings', in Patricia D'Antonio, Julie A. Fairman and Jean C. Whelan (eds), *Routledge Handbook on the Global History of Nursing* (London: Routledge, 2013)

Cooper, Joanne E., 'Shaping meaning: Women's diaries, journals and letters – the old and the new', *Women's Studies International Forum* 10, 1 (1987): 95–9.

Cooter, Roger, and Sturdy, Steve, 'Of war, medicine and modernity', in Roger

Cooter, Mark Harrison and Steve Sturdy (eds), *Medicine and Modern Warfare* (Amsterdam: Rodopi, 1998).

Costello, John, *Love, Sex and War: Changing Values 1939–45* (London: Collins, 1985).

Cowman, Krista, and Jackson, Louise A., 'Middle-class women and professional identity', *Women's History Review* 14, 2 (2005): 165–79.

Crang, Jeremy A., '"Come into the Army Maud": Women, military conscription, and the Markham Inquiry', *Defence Studies* 8, 3 (2008): 381–95.

Crew, F.A.E., *The Army Medical Services: Volume I: Administration* (London: HMSO, 1953).

Crew, F.A.E., *The Army Medical Services: Volume II: Campaigns: Hong Kong, Malaya, Iceland and the Faroes, Libya, 1942–1943, North West Africa* (London: HMSO, 1957).

Crew, F.A.E., 'The Army medical services', in Arthur Salusbury MacNalty and W. Franklin Mellor (eds), *Medical Services in War: The Principal Medical Lessons of the Second World War* (London: HMSO, 1968).

Dale, Charlotte, 'Traversing the veldt with "Tommy Atkins": The clinical challenges of nursing typhoid patients during the Second Anglo-Boer War (1899–1902)', in Jane Brooks and Christine E. Hallett (eds), *One Hundred Years of Wartime Nursing Practices, 1854–1953* (Manchester: Manchester University Press, 2015).

Dale, Charlotte, 'The social exploits and behaviour of nurses during the Anglo-Boer War, 1899–1902', in Helen Sweet and Sue Hawkins (eds), *Colonial Caring: A History of Colonial and Post-Colonial Nursing* (Manchester: Manchester University Press, 2015).

Das, Santanu, *Touch and Intimacy in First World War Literature* (Cambridge: Cambridge University Press, 2005).

Davidoff, Leonore, *Worlds Between: Historical Perspectives on Gender and Class* (Cambridge: Polity Press, 1995).

Davin, Anna, 'Imperialism and motherhood', *History Workshop Journal* 5 (1978): 9–65.

DeGroot, Gerard J., '"Lipstick on her nipples, cordite in her hair": Sex and romance among British servicewomen during the Second World War', in Gerard J. DeGroot and Corinna Peniston-Bird, *A Soldier and a Woman* (Abingdon: Taylor and Francis, 2014).

DiCenzo, Maria, '"Our Freedom and its Results": Measuring progress in the aftermath of suffrage', *Women's History Review* 23, 3 (2014): 421–40.

Dickinson, Tommy, *'Curing Queers': Mental Nurses and their Patients, 1935–74* (Manchester: Manchester University Press, 2015).

Dingwall, Robert, Rafferty, Anne Marie, and Webster, Charles, *An Introduction to the Social History of Nursing* (London: Routledge, 1988).

Dixon Vuic, Kara, '"Officer, nurse, woman": Army Nurse Corps recruitment for the Vietnam War', *Nursing History Review* 14 (2006): 111–59.

Dixon Vuic, Kara, *Officer, Nurse, Woman: The Army Nurse Corps in the Vietnam War* (Baltimore, MD: Johns Hopkins University Press, 2010, Kindle edition).

Dixon Vuic, Kara, 'Wartime nursing and power', in Patricia D'Antonio, Julie A. Fairman and Jean C. Whelan (eds), *Routledge Handbook on the Global History of Nursing* (London: Routledge, 2013).

Doughty, Dorothy B., 'History of ostomy surgery', *Journal of Wound Ostomy Continence Nursing* 35,1 (2008): 34–8.

Dyhouse, Carol, 'Women students and the London Medical Schools, 1914–39: The anatomy of a masculine culture', *Gender and History* 10, 1 (1998): 110–32.

Dyhouse, Carol, 'Troubled identities: gender and status in the history of the mixed college in English universities since 1945', *Women's History Review* 12, 2 (2006) 169–94.

Easingwood, Ruth, '"I was merely a shorthand typist": British women at work in the British zone of occupied Germany, 1945–1949', *Women's History Magazine* 67 (2011): 20–7.

Enloe, Cynthia, *Does Khaki Become You? The Militarization of Women's Lives* (London: Pandora, 1988).

Evans, Richard J., *The Third Reich at War* (London: Penguin, 2009).

Fairman, Julie, 'Alterative visions: the nurse-technology relationship in the context of the history of technology', *Nursing History Review* 6 (1998): 129–46.

Fairman, Julie, and D'Antonio, Patricia, 'Virtual power: Gendering the nurse-technology relationship', *Nursing Inquiry* 6, 3 (1999): 178–86.

Fairman, Julie, and D'Antonio, Patricia, 'Reimagining nursing's place in the history of clinical practice', *Journal of the History of Medicine and Allied Health Sciences* 63, 4 (2008): 435–46.

Fairman, Julie, and Lynaugh, Joan E., *Critical Care Nursing: A History* (Philadelphia, PA: University of Pennsylvania Press, 1998).

Fennell, Jonathan, 'Courage and cowardice in the North African Campaign: The Eighth Army and defeat in the summer of 1942', *War in History* 20,1 (2013): 99–122.

Finlay, Adrianne, 'Cherry Ames, disembodied nurse: War sexuality, and sacrifice in the novels of Helen Wells', *The Journal of Popular Culture* 43, 6 (2010): 1189–206.

Flanagan, Ben, and Bloxham, Donald (eds), *Remembering Belsen: Eyewitnesses Record the Liberation* (London: Vallentine Mitchell, 2005).

Fletcher, Angharad, 'Sisters behind the wire: Reappraising Australian military nursing and internment in the Pacific during World War II', *Medical History* 55 (2011): 419–24.

Flynn, Karen, 'Proletarianization, professionalization and Caribbean immigrant nurses', *Canadian Woman Studies* 18, 1 (1998): 57–60.

Fussell, Paul, *Wartime: Understanding and Behavior in the Second World War* (New York: Oxford University Press, 1989).

Gilbert, Martin, *The Second World War: A Complete History* (London: Phoenix, 2009).

Gilmour, Jean A., 'Hybrid space: Constituting the hospitals as a home space for patients', *Nursing Inquiry* 13, 1 (2006): 16–22.

Goodman, Phil, '"Patriotic femininity": Women's morals and men's morale during the Second World War', *Gender and History* 10, 2 (1998): 278–93.

Gottlieb, Julie V., 'Munich by-elections, 1938–1939', in Julie V. Gottlieb and Richard Toye, *The Aftermath of Suffrage: Women, Gender, and Politics in Britain 1918–1945* (Basingstoke: Palgrave Macmillan, 2013).

Gottlieb, Julie V., and Toye, Richard, *The Aftermath of Suffrage: Women, Gender, and Politics in Britain 1918–1945* (Basingstoke: Palgrave Macmillan, 2013).

Grayzel, Susan R., '"Fighting for the idea of home life": *Mrs Miniver* and Anglo-American representations of domestic morale', in Philippa Levine and Susan R. Grayzel (eds), *Gender, Labour, War and Empire* (London: Palgrave Macmillan, 2009).

Grayzel, Susan R., *At Home and Under Fire: Air Raids and Culture in Britain from the Great War to the Blitz* (Cambridge: Cambridge University Press, 2012).

Greenberg, M., 'Therapeutic play: Developing humor in the nurse–patient relationship', *Journal of the New York State Nurses Association* 34, 1 (2003): 25–31.

Gregg, Alan, 'Adaptation of survival: Reflections on our postwar problems', *American Journal of Nursing* 44, 10 (1944): 923–7.

Gubar, Susan, '"This is my rifle, this is my gun": World War II and the blitz on women', in Margaret Randolph Higonnet, Jane Jenson, Sonya Michel and Margaret Collins Weitz (eds), *Behind the Lines: Gender and the Two World Wars* (New Haven, CT: Yale University Press, 1987).

Hadley Jackson, Margaret, 'Causes and significance of the dwindling family', in Sir James Marchant (ed.), *Rebuilding Family Life in the Post-War World: An Enquiry with Recommendations* (London: Odhams Press, 1945).

Haggart, Ali, '"Desperate housewives" and the domestic environment in post-war Britain: Individual perspectives', *Oral History* 37, 1 (2009): 53–60.

Hall, Martha L., Orzada, Belinda T., and Lopez-Gydosh, Dilia, 'American women's wartime dress: Sociocultural ambiguities regarding women's roles during World War II', *The Journal of American Culture* 38, 3 (2015): 232–42.

Hallam, Julia, *Nursing the Image: Media, Culture and Professional Identity* (London: Routledge, 2000).

Hallett, Christine E., 'The personal writings of First World War nurses: A study of the interplay of authorial intention and scholarly interpretation', *Nursing Inquiry* 14, 4 (2007): 320–9.

Hallett, Christine E., *Containing Trauma: Nursing Work in the First World War* (Manchester: Manchester University Press, 2009).

Hallett, Christine E., *Veiled Warriors: Allied Nurses of the First World War* (Oxford: Oxford University Press, 2014).

Hallett, Christine E., '"This fiendish mode of warfare": Nursing the victims of gas poisoning in the First World War', in Jane Brooks and Christine E. Hallett (eds), *One Hundred Years of Wartime Nursing Practices, 1854–1953* (Manchester: Manchester University Press, 2015).

Hallett, Christine E., *Nurse Writers of the Great War* (Manchester: Manchester University Press, 2016).

Hardman, Leslie, and Goodman, Cecily, *The Survivors: The Story of the Belsen Remnant* (London: Vallentine Mitchell, 2009).

Harris, Kirsty, *More than Bombs and Bandages: Australian Army Nurses at Work in World War I* (Newport: Big Sky Publishing, 2011, Kindle edition).

Harris, Kirsty, '"Health, healing and harmony": Invalid cookery and feeding by Australian nurses in the Middle East in the First World War', in Jane Brooks and Christine E. Hallett (eds), *One Hundred Years of Wartime Nursing Practices, 1854–1953* (Manchester: Manchester University Press, 2015).

Harrison, Mark, 'The medicalization of war – the militarization of medicine', *The Society for the Social History of Medicine* 9, 2 (1996): 267–76.

Harrison, Mark, *Medicine and Victory: British Military Medicine in the Second World War* (Oxford: Oxford University Press, 2004).

Harrison, Mark, *The Medical War: British Military Medicine in the First World War* (Oxford: Oxford University Press, 2010).

Hawkins, Sue, *Nursing and Women's Labour in the Nineteenth Century: The Quest for Independence* (London: Routledge, 2010).

Hay, Ian, *One Hundred Years of Army Nursing: The Story of the British Army Nursing Services from the Time of Florence Nightingale to the Present Day* (London: Cassell, 1953).

Helmstadter, Carol, 'Class, gender and professional expertise: British military nursing in the Crimean War', in Jane Brooks and Christine E. Hallett (eds), *One Hundred Years of Wartime Nursing Practices, 1854–1953* (Manchester: Manchester University Press, 2015).

Henderson, Virginia, *The Nature of Nursing: Reflections after 25 Years* (New York: National League for Nursing Press, 1991).

Higonnet, Margaret Randolph, and Higonnet, Patrice L.-R., 'The double helix', in Margaret Randolph Higonnet, Jane Jenson, Sonya Michel and Margaret Collins Weitz (eds), *Behind the Lines: Gender and the Two World Wars* (New Haven, CT: Yale University Press,1987).

Higonnet, Margaret Randolph, Jenson, Jane, Michel, Sonya, and Weitz, Margaret Collins, 'Introduction', in Margaret Randolph Higonnet, Jane Jenson, Sonya Michel and Margaret Collins Weitz (eds), *Behind the Lines: Gender and the Two World Wars* (New Haven, CT: Yale University Press,1987).

Higonnet, Margaret Randolph, Jenson, Jane, Michel, Sonya, and Weitz, Margaret Collins (eds), *Behind the Lines: Gender and the Two World Wars* (New Haven, CT: Yale University Press, 1987).

Honey, Maureen, *Creating Rosie the Riveter: Class, Gender, and Propaganda during World War II* (Amherst, MA: University of Massachusetts Press, 1984).

Howell, Jessica, Rafferty, Anne Marie, and Snaith, Anna, '(Author)ity abroad: The life writing of colonial nurses', *International Journal of Nursing Studies* 48 (2011): 1155–62.

Howell, Jessica, Rafferty, Anne Marie, Wall, Rosemary, and Snaith, Anna, 'Nursing the tropics: Nurses as agents of imperial hygiene', *Journal of Public Health* 35, 2 (2013): 338–41.

Jackson, Angela, 'Blood and guts: Nursing with the International Brigades in the Spanish Civil War, 1936–39', in Jane Brooks and Christine E. Hallett (eds), *One Hundred Years of Nursing Wartime Practices, 1854–1953* (Manchester: Manchester University Press, 2015).

Jalland, Pat, 'A culture of silent grief? The transformation of bereavement care in 20th century England', *Bereavement Care* 32, 1 (2013): 16–22.

Jones, Edgar, and Wessely, Simon, 'Psychiatric battle casualties: An intra- and interwar comparison', *The British Journal of Psychiatry* 178 (2001): 242–7.

Justham, David, '"Those maggots – they did a wonderful job": The nurses' role in wound management in civilian hospitals during the Second World War', in Jane Brooks and Christine E. Hallett (eds), *One Hundred Years of Nursing Wartime Practices, 1854–1953* (Manchester: Manchester University Press, 2015).

Kenyon, Olga, *800 Years of Women's Letters* (Stroud: Alan Sutton Publishing, 1992).

Khan, Yasmin, 'Sex in an imperial war zone: Transnational encounters in Second World War India', *History Workshop Journal* 73 (2012): 241–58.

Kushner, Tony, 'The memory of Belsen', in Jo Reilly, David Cesarani, Tony Kushner and Colin Richmond (eds), *Belsen in History and Memory* (London: Frank Cass, 1997).

Laffin, John, *Women in Battle* (London: Abelard Schuman, 1967).

Lamb, M.M., 'Nursing is what?', *International Nursing Review* 17 (1970): 373–80.

Lawler, Jocalyn, *Behind the Screens: Nursing, Somology and the Problem of the Body* (Melbourne: Churchill Livingstone, 1991).

Lewenson, Sandra B., 'Doing historical research', Sandra B. Lewenson and Eleanor Krohn Herrmann (eds), *Capturing Nursing History: A Guide to Historical Methods in Research* (New York: Springer, 2008).

Lewenson, Sandra B., and Krohn Herrmann, Eleanor (eds), *Capturing Nursing History: A Guide to Historical Methods in Research* (New York: Springer, 2008).

Linker, Beth, *War's Waste: Rehabilitation in World War I America* (Chicago: University of Chicago Press, 2011).

Lockertsen, Jan Thore, Fause, Ashild, Hallett, Christine E., and Brooks, Jane, 'The Norwegian Mobile Army Surgical Hospital: Nursing at the front', in Jane Brooks and Christine E. Hallett (eds), *One Hundred Years of Nursing Wartime Practices, 1854–1953* (Manchester: Manchester University Press, 2015).

Lucas, James, *War in the Desert: The Eighth Army at El Alamein* (London: Arms and Armour Press, 1982).

McBryde, Brenda, *Quiet Heroines: Nurses of the Second World War* (London: Chatto and Windus, 1985).

McEwan, Ian, *Atonement* (London: Vintage Books, 2002).

McGann, Susan, *The Battle of the Nurses* (Middlesex: Scutari Press, 1992).

MacGuire, Jillian, 'Tailoring research for therapeutic nursing practice', in Richard McMahon and Alan Pearson, *Nursing as Therapy* (2nd edn) (Cheltenham: Stanley Thornes, 1998).

McIntosh, Jean, and Dingwall, Robert, 'Teamwork in theory and practice', in Robert Dingwall and Jean McIntosh (eds), *Readings in the Sociology of Nursing* (Edinburgh: Churchill Livingstone, 1978).

MacNalty, Arthur Salusbury, 'Medical research', in Arthur Salusbury MacNalty and W. Franklin Mellor (eds), *Medical Services in War: The Principal Medical Lessons of the Second World War* (London: HMSO, 1968).

MacNalty, Arthur Salusbury, and Mellor, W. Franklin (eds), *Medical Services in War: The Principal Medical Lessons of the Second World War* (London: HMSO, 1968).

Mackie, Mary, *Sky Wards: A History of the Princess Mary's Royal Air Force Nursing Service* (London: Robert Hale, 2001).

McMahon, Richard, 'Therapeutic nursing: Theory, issues and practice', in Richard McMahon and Alan Pearson, *Nursing as Therapy* (2nd edn) (Cheltenham: Stanley Thornes, 1998).

McPherson, Kathryn, *Bedside Matters: The Transformation of Canadian Nursing, 1900–1990* (Toronto: Oxford University Press Canada, 1996).

Marwick, Arthur, *The New Nature of History: Knowledge, Evidence, Language* (Basingstoke: Palgrave, 2001).

Mayhew, Emily, *The Reconstruction of Warriors: Archibald McIndoe, The Royal Air Force and the Guinea Pig Club* (Barnsley: Greenhill Books, 2010, Kindle edition).

Meehan, Therese Connell, 'Careful nursing: A model for contemporary nursing practice', *Journal of Advanced Nursing*, 44, 1 (2003): 99–107.

Meyer, Leisa D., *Creating GI Jane: Sexuality and Power in the Women's Army Corps During World War II* (New York: Columbia University Press, 1996).

Minister of Health, Secretary of State for Scotland and the Minister of Labour and National Service, 'Staffing the hospitals: An urgent national need', *International History of Nursing Journal* 3, 3 (1998): 15. Reprinted from pamphlet, Minister of Health, Secretary of State for Scotland and the Minister of Labour and National Service, 'Staffing the hospitals: An urgent national need' (London: HMSO, 1945) RCN Archives, Pamphlet Collection 11AD, RCN Archives, Edinburgh.

Moeller, Robert G., 'What did you do in the war, *mutti*? Courageous women, compassionate commanders and stories of the Second World War', *German History* 22, 4 (2004): 563–94.

Montgomerie, Deborah, 'Assessing Rosie: World War II, New Zealand women and the iconography of femininity', *Gender and History*, 8, 1 (1996): 108–32.

Moore, Jeanne, 'Placing the home in context', *Journal of Environmental Psychology* 20 (2000): 207–17.

Mortimer, Barbara, *Sisters: Extraordinary True-Life Stories from Nurses in World War Two* (London: Hutchinson, 2012).

Nestel, Sheryl, '(Ad)ministering angels: Colonial nursing and the extension of empire in Africa', *Journal of Medical Humanities* 19, 4 (1998): 257–77.

Neushul, Peter, 'Fighting research: Army participation in the clinical testing and mass production of penicillin during the Second World War', in Roger Cooter, Mark Harrison and Steve Sturdy (eds), *War, Medicine and Modernity* (Stroud: Sutton Publishing, 1998).

Newlands, Emma, *Civilians into Soldiers: War, the Body and British Army Recruits, 1939–45* (Manchester: Manchester University Press, 2014).

Noakes, Lucy, *War and the British: Gender, Memory and National Identity* (London: I.B. Tauris, 1998).

Noakes, Lucy, *Women in the British Army: War and the Gentle Sex, 1907–1948* (London, Routledge, 2006, Kindle edition).

Noakes, Lucy, '"Serve to save": Gender, citizenship and Civil Defence in Britain, 1937–41', *Journal of Contemporary History* 47, 4 (2012): 734–53.

Noakes, Lucy, '"Gentle in manner, resolute in deed": Women and the British army in the post-war years', *Women's History Magazine* 76 (Autumn 2014): 5–12.

Norman, Elizabeth M., and Eifried, Sharon, 'How did they all survive? An analysis of American nurses' experiences in Japanese Prisoner-of-War camps', *Nursing History Review* 3 (1995): 105–27.

Ondaatje, Michael, *The English Patient* (London: Bloomsbury, 1992).

Parry, Joyce Ffoulkes, *Joyce's War: The Second World War Journal of a Queen Alexandra's Imperial Military Nursing Service Nurse*, ed. Rhiannon Evans (Stroud: The History Press, 2015, Kindle edition).

Pattinson, Juliette, '"Playing the daft lassie with them": Gender, captivity and the Special Operations Executive during the Second World War', *European Review of History* 13, 2 (2006): 271–92.

Pattinson, Juliette, *Behind Enemy Lines: Gender, Passing and the Special Operations Executive in the Second World War* (Manchester: Manchester University Press, 2007).

Peniston-Bird, Corinna, 'Classifying the body in the Second World War: British men in and out of uniform', *Body and Society* 9, 4 (2003): 31–48.

Perks, Robert, and Thomson, Alastair, *The Oral History Reader* (London: Routledge, 1998).

Piggott, Juliet, *Queen Alexandra's Royal Army Nursing Corps* (London: Leo Cooper, 1975).

Poovey, Mary, *Uneven Developments: The Ideological Work of Gender in Mid-Victorian England* (Chicago: University of Chicago Press, 1988).

Porter, Dorothy, *Health, Civilization and the State: A History of Public Health from Ancient to Modern Times* (London: Routledge, 1999).

Purvis, June, 'Using primary sources when researching women's history from a feminist perspective', *Women's History Review* 1, 2 (1992): 273–306.

Rae, Ruth, *Scarlet Poppies: The Army Experience of Australian Nurses during World War I* (Burwood: College of Nursing, 2004).

Rafferty, Anne Marie, *The Politics of Nursing Knowledge* (London: Routledge, 1996).

Reilly, Jo, Cesarani, David, Kushner, Tony, and Richmond, Colin (eds), *Belsen in History and Memory* (London: Frank Cass, 1997).

Reilly, Jo, 'Cleaner, carer and occasional dance partner? Writing women back into the liberation of Bergen-Belsen', in Jo Reilly, David Cesarani, Tony Kushner and Colin Richmond (eds), *Belsen in History and Memory* (London: Frank Cass, 1997).

Richardson, Sharon L., '"Stand up and be counted": Nursing at the Calgary General Hospital after the Second World War', *Canadian Bulletin of Medical History* 18 (2001): 297–323.

Rickard, Wendy, 'Oral history – "More dangerous than therapy"? Interviewees' reflections on recording traumatic or taboo issues', *Oral History* 26, 2, 'Memory, Trauma and Ethics' (1998): 34–48.

Rogers, Anna, *While You're Away: New Zealand Nurses at War, 1899–1948* (Auckland: Auckland University Press 2003).

Roper, Michael, 'Between Manliness and Masculinity: The "War" Generation" and the Psychology of Fear in Britain, 1914–1950', *Journal of British Studies* 44 (2005): 343–62.

Rose, Sonya O., *Which People's War? National Identity and Citizenship in Britain, 1939–1945* (Oxford: Oxford University Press, 2003, Kindle edition).

Rowbotham, Sheila, *A Century of Women: A History of Women in Britain and the United States* (London: Penguin, 1999).

Sandelowski, Margarete, 'Venous envy: The post-World War II debate over IV nursing', *Advances in Nursing Science* 22, 1 (1999): 52–62.

Sandelowski, Margarete, *Devices and Desires: Gender, Technology and American Nursing* (Chapel Hill, NC: University of North Carolina Press, 2000).

Sangster, Joan, '"Telling our stories": Feminist debates and the use of oral history', *Women's History Review* 3, 1 (1994): 5–28.

Sarkar, Mahua, 'Between craft and method: Meaning and inter-subjectivity in oral history analysis', *Journal of Historical Sociology* 25, 4 (2012): 578–600.

Sarnecky, Mary, *A History of the US Army Nurse Corps* (Philadelphia, PA: University of Pennsylvania Press, 1999).

Schultz, Jane E., *Women at the Front: Hospital Workers in Civil War America* (Chapel Hill, NC: University of North Carolina Press, 2004).

Shephard, Ben, *After Daybreak: The Liberation of Belsen, 1945* (London: Pimlico, 2005).

Shephard, Ben, 'The medical relief at Belsen', in Suzanne Bardgett and David Cesarani (eds), *Belsen 1945, New Historical Perspectives* (London: Vallentine Mitchell, 2006).

Shkimba, M., and Flynn, Karen, '"In England we did nursing": Caribbean and British nurses in Great Britain and Canada, 1950–70', in Barbara Mortimer and Susan McGann (eds), *New Directions in Nursing History: International Perspectives* (London: Routledge, 2004).

Sintos Coloma, Roland, '"White gazes, brown breasts": Imperial feminism and disciplining desires and bodies in colonial encounters', *Paedagogica Historica: International Journal of the History of Education* 48, 2 (2012): 243–61.

Sixsmith, Judith, 'The meaning of home: An exploratory study of environmental experience', *Journal of Environmental Psychology* 6 (1986): 281–98.

Smith, Harold, 'The effect of the war on the status of women', in Harold Smith (ed.), *War and Social Change: British Society in the Second World War* (Manchester: Manchester University Press, 1986).

Smyth, John, *The Will to Live: The Story of Dame Margot Turner* (London: Hills and Lacy, 1970)

Solano, Diana, and Rafferty, Anne Marie, 'Can lessons be learned from history? The origins of the British imperial nurse labour market: A discussion paper', *International Journal of Nursing Studies* 44, 6 (2007): 1055–63.

Starns, Penny, 'Fighting militarism? British nursing during the Second World War', in Roger Cooter, Mark Harrison and Steve Sturdy (eds), *War, Medicine and Modernity* (Stroud: Sutton Publishing, 1998).

Starns, Penny, *Nurses at War: Women on the Frontline, 1939–45* (Stroud: Sutton Publishing, 2000).

Starns, Penny, *Surviving Tenko: The Story of Margot Turner* (Stroud: The History Press, 2010).

Summerfield, Penny, 'What women learned from the Second World War', *History of Education* 18, 3 (1989): 213–29.

Summerfield, Penny, 'Women and war in the twentieth century', in June Purvis (ed.), *Women's History: Britain, 1850–1945* (London: UCL Press, 1995).

Summerfield, Penny, 'Gender and war in the twentieth century', *The International History Review* 19, 1 (1997): 3–15.

Summerfield, Penny, *Reconstructing Women's Wartime Lives: Discourse and Subjectivity in Oral Histories of the Second World War* (Manchester: Manchester University Press, 1998).

Summerfield, Penny, '"They didn't want women back in that job": The Second World War and the construction of gendered work histories', *Labour History Review* 63, 1 (1998): 83–104.

Summerfield, Penny, 'Culture and composure: Creating narratives of the gendered self in oral history interviews', *Cultural and Social History* 1 (2004): 65–93.

Summerfield, Penny, and Peniston-Bird, Corinna, 'Women in the firing-line: The

Home Guard and the defence of gender boundaries in Britain in the Second World War', *Women's History Review* 9, 2 (2000): 231–55.

Summers, Anne, *Angels and Citizens: British Women as Military Nurses, 1854–1914* (Newbury: Threshold Press, 2000).

Sumners, Ann D., 'Professional nurses attitudes towards humour', *Journal of Advanced Nursing* 15 (1999): 194–200.

Sweet, Helen M., and Dougall, Rona, *Community Nursing and Primary Healthcare in Twentieth-Century Britain* (New York: Routledge, 2008).

Tanay, Mary Anne Lagmay, Roberts, Julia and Ream, Emma, 'Humour in adult cancer care: A concept analysis', *Journal of Advanced Nursing* 69, 9 (2012): 2131–40.

Taylor, Beverley, 'Ordinariness in nursing as therapy', in Richard McMahon and Alan Pearson, *Nursing as Therapy* (2nd edn) (Cheltenham: Stanley Thornes, 1998).

Taylor, Eric, *Women Who Went to War, 1938–46* (London: Robert Hale, 1988).

Taylor, Eric, *Front-Line Nurse: British Nurses in World War II* (London: Robert Hale, 1997).

Taylor, Eric, *Combat Nurse* (London: Robert Hale, 1999).

Taylor, Eric, *Wartime Nurse: 100 years from the Crimea to Korea 1854–1954* (London: Robert Hale, 2001).

Tesseyman, Sheri, 'Complex alliance: A study of relationships between nursing and medicine in Britain and the United States of America, 1860–1914' [unpublished PhD] (Manchester: University of Manchester, 2013).

Terraine, John, 'Christmas 1914, and after', *History Today* 29 (1979): 781–9.

Thane, Pat, 'What difference did the vote make? Women in public and private life in Britain since 1918', *Historical Research* 76, 192 (2003): 268–85.

Thane, Pat, 'Family life and "normality" in postwar British culture', in Richard Bessel and Dirk Schumann (eds), *Life after Death: Approaches to a Cultural and Social History of Europe during the 1940s and 1950s* (Cambridge: Cambridge University Press, 2003).

Thane, Pat, 'Girton Graduates: earning and learning, 1920s–1980s', *Women's History Review* 13, 3 (2004): 347–61.

Thompson, Paul, *The Voice of the Past: Oral History* (Oxford: Oxford University Press, 2000).

Thurgood, Graham J., 'Nurses' voices from the archives', *Journal of the Society of Archivists* 31, 2 (2010): 135–47.

Toman, Cynthia, 'Blood work: Canadian nursing and blood transfusion, 1942–1990', *Nursing History Review* 9 (2001): 51–78.

Toman, Cynthia, '"Body work": Nurses and the delegation of medical technology at the Ottawa Civic Hospital, 1947-1972', *Canadian Journal of the History of Science, Technology and Medicine* 29, 2 (2006): 155–75.

Toman, Cynthia, *An Officer and a Lady: Canadian Military Nursing and the Second World War* (Vancouver: University of British Columbia Press, 2007).

Toman, Cynthia, 'Front lines and frontiers: War as legitimate work for nurses, 1939–1945', *Social History* 40, 79 (2007): 45–74.

Toman, Cynthia, *Sister Soldiers of the Great War: The Nurses of the Canadian Army Medical Corps* (Vancouver: University of British Columbia Press, 2016).

Tosh, John, *The Pursuit of History* (London: Longman, 2002).

Travelbee, Joyce, *Interpersonal Aspects of Nursing* (Philadelphia, PA: F.A. Davis, 1971).

Traynor, Michael, Boland, Maggie, and Buus, Niels, 'Autonomy, evidence and intuition: Nurses and decision-making', *Journal of Advanced Nursing* 66, 7 (2010): 1584–91.

Twells, Alison, '"Went into raptures": Reading emotion in the ordinary wartime diary, 1941–1946', *Women's History Review* 25, 1 (2016): 143–60.

Twomey, Christina, 'Australian nurse POWs: Gender, war and captivity', *Australian Historical Studies* 36, 124 (2004): 255–74.

Twomey, Christina, 'Double displacement: Western nurses return home from Japanese internment camps in Second World War', *Gender and History* 21, 3 (2009): 670–84.

Tyrer, Nicola, *Sisters in Arms: British Army Nurses Tell their Story* (London: Phoenix, 2008).

Valley, Myra, 'The training of "Agents of Empire": Educational and early career patterns for Scottish nurses of the Colonial and Overseas Nursing Associations, 1899–1939', *The Bulletin of the UK Association for the History of Nursing*, 3 (2014): 57–72.

Vicinus, Martha, *Independent Women: Work and Community for Single Women, 1850–1920* (London: Virago, 1985).

Vickery, Amanda, 'Historiographical review: Golden age to separate spheres? A review of the categories and chronology of English women's history', *The Historical Journal* 36, 2 (1993): 383–414.

Walby, Sylvia, and Greenwell, June, *Medicine and Nursing: Professions in a Changing Health Service* (London: Sage, 1994).

Warner, Lavinia, and Sandilands, John, *Women Beyond the Wire: A Story of Prisoners of the Japanese, 1942–45* (London: Michael Joseph, 1982).

Watson, Janet S.K., 'Khaki girls, VADs, and Tommy's sister: Gender and class in First World War Britain', *The International History Review* 19, 1 (1997): 32–50.

Watson, Janet S.K., 'Wars in the wards: The social construction of medical work in First World War Britain', *Journal of British Studies* 41, 4 (2002): 484–510.

Watson, Janet S.K., *Fighting Different Wars: Experience, Memory, and the First World War in Britain* (Cambridge, Cambridge University Press, 2007).

Webster, Charles, 'Nursing as the early crisis of the NHS', *International History of Nursing Journal* 3, 3 (1998): 36–43.

Webster, Charles, *The National Health Service: A Political History* (Oxford: Oxford University Press, 2002).

Whitehead, Ian, 'The British medical officer on the Western Front', in Roger

Cooter, Mark Harrison, and Steve Sturdy (eds), *Medicine and Modern Warfare* (Amsterdam: Rodopi, 1999).

Willmot, Louise, 'Women and resistance', in Gilly Carr, Paul Sanders and Louise Willmot (eds), *Protest, Defiance and Resistance in the Channel Islands German Occupation, 1940–45* (London: Bloomsbury, 2014).

Yap, Felicia, 'Voices and silence of memory: Civilian internees of the Japanese in British Asia during the Second World War', *Journal of British Studies* 50 (October 2011): 917–40.

Yap, Felicia, 'Creativity and the body: Civilian internees in British Asia in the Second World War', in Gilly Carr and Harold Mytum (eds), *Cultural Heritage and Prisoners of War: Creativity Behind Barbed Wire* (London: Routledge, 2012).

Zweiniger-Bargielowska, Ina, 'Housewifery', in Ina Zweiniger-Bargielowska (ed.), *Women in the Twentieth-Century* (Harlow: Pearson Education, 2001).

Index

Page numbers in **bold** refer to figures

EU authorised representative for GPSR:
Easy Access System Europe, Mustamäe tee 50,
10621 Tallinn, Estonia
gpsr.requests@easproject.com

www.ingramcontent.com/pod-product-compliance
Ingram Content Group UK Ltd.
Pitfield, Milton Keynes, MK11 3LW, UK
UKHW021833100926
8556IPUK00004B/324
9781526119063